Child Injury
and the Determinants of Health

Child Injury
and the Determinants of Health

Editors

Amy Peden
Richard Franklin

MDPI • Basel • Beijing • Wuhan • Barcelona • Belgrade • Manchester • Tokyo • Cluj • Tianjin

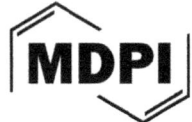

Editors
Amy Peden
School of Population Health,
University of New South Wales
Australia

Richard Franklin
Department of Public Health
and Tropical Medicine,
College of Public Health,
Medical and Veterinary Sciences,
James Cook University
Australia

Editorial Office
MDPI
St. Alban-Anlage 66
4052 Basel, Switzerland

This is a reprint of articles from the Special Issue published online in the open access journal *Children* (ISSN 2227-9067) (available at: https://www.mdpi.com/journal/children/special_issues/Child_Injury).

For citation purposes, cite each article independently as indicated on the article page online and as indicated below:

LastName, A.A.; LastName, B.B.; LastName, C.C. Article Title. *Journal Name* **Year**, *Volume Number*, Page Range.

ISBN 978-3-0365-0600-5 (Hbk)
ISBN 978-3-0365-0601-2 (PDF)

Cover image courtesy of Nasik Lababan.

© 2021 by the authors. Articles in this book are Open Access and distributed under the Creative Commons Attribution (CC BY) license, which allows users to download, copy and build upon published articles, as long as the author and publisher are properly credited, which ensures maximum dissemination and a wider impact of our publications.

The book as a whole is distributed by MDPI under the terms and conditions of the Creative Commons license CC BY-NC-ND.

Contents

About the Editors vii

Amy E. Peden and Richard C. Franklin
Child Injury Prevention: It Is Time to Address the Determinants of Health
Reprinted from: *Children* 2021, 8, 46, doi:10.3390/children8010046 1

Medhavi Gupta, Sujoy Roy, Ranjan Panda, Pompy Konwar and Jagnoor Jagnoor
Interventions for Child Drowning Reduction in the Indian Sundarbans: Perspectives from the Ground
Reprinted from: *Children* 2020, 7, 291, doi:10.3390/children7120291 5

Jonathan P. Guevarra, Amy E. Peden, Lita L. Orbillo, Maria Rosario Sylvia Z. Uy, Joseph John R. Madrilejos, John Juliard L. Go, Rammell Eric C. Martinez, Lolita L. Cavinta and Richard C Franklin
Preventing Child Drowning in the Philippines: The Need to Address the Determinants of Health
Reprinted from: *Children* 2021, 8, 29, doi:10.3390/children8010029 23

Isabell Sakamoto, Sarah Stempski, Vijay Srinivasan, Tien Le, Elizabeth Bennett and Linda Quan
Adolescent Water Safety Behaviors, Skills, Training and Their Association with Risk-Taking Behaviors and Risk and Protective Factors
Reprinted from: *Children* 2020, 7, 301, doi:10.3390/children7120301 43

Amy E. Peden and Richard C. Franklin
Exploring the Impact of Remoteness and Socio-Economic Status on Child and Adolescent Injury-Related Mortality in Australia
Reprinted from: *Children* 2021, 8, 5, doi:10.3390/children8010005 57

Keira Bury, Jonine Jancey and Justine E. Leavy
Parent Mobile Phone Use in Playgrounds: A Paradox of Convenience
Reprinted from: *Children* 2020, 7, 284, doi:10.3390/children7120284 77

Rebbecca Lilley, Bronwen McNoe, Gabrielle Davie, Brandon de Graaf and Tim Driscoll
Work-Related Fatalities Involving Children in New Zealand, 1999–2014
Reprinted from: *Children* 2021, 8, 4, doi:10.3390/children8010004 89

Alexandra Mihaela Stoica, Oana Elena Stoica, Ramona Elena Vlad, Anca Maria Pop and Monica Monea
The Correlation between Oral Self-Harm and Ethnicity in Institutionalized Children
Reprinted from: *Children* 2021, 8, 2, doi:10.3390/children8010002 101

Josip Karuc, Mario Jelčić, Maroje Sorić, Marjeta Mišigoj-Duraković and Goran Marković
Does Sex Dimorphism Exist in Dysfunctional Movement Patterns during the Sensitive Period of Adolescence?
Reprinted from: *Children* 2020, 7, 308, doi:10.3390/children7120308 111

Damir Sekulic, Dasa Prus, Ante Zevrnja, Mia Peric and Petra Zaletel
Predicting Injury Status in Adolescent Dancers Involved in Different Dance Styles: A Prospective Study
Reprinted from: *Children* 2020, 7, 297, doi:10.3390/children7120297 121

Junya Saeki, Satoshi Iizuka, Hiroaki Sekino, Ayahiro Suzuki, Toshihiro Maemichi and Suguru Torii
Optimum Angle of Force Production Temporarily Changes Due to Growth in Male Adolescence
Reprinted from: *Children* **2021**, *8*, 20, doi:10.3390/children8010020 . . . . **135**

About the Editors

Amy Peden has extensive experience in injury prevention research, policy and practice, having worked in the field for 13 years. Dr Peden's work focuses on drowning prevention and she is passionate about reducing injury burden in rural and remote communities. Her other areas of focus include the impact of alcohol on injury risk, improving data quality and science communication.

Richard Franklin is a pracademic who uses an evidence-based approach to developing real-world solutions to improve safety, health and wellbeing. His work focuses on child safety, health systems, drowning prevention, farm safety, road safety, trauma, alcohol impact, falls, the safety of older people, first aid, disasters and resilience, with a focus on those living in rural areas and the tropics. He is an epidemiologist who uses a mixed-methods approach to addressing real-world problems using a wide range of data collection methods including big data, data linkage, interviews, focus groups, surveys, program evaluation, produce evaluation, surveillance, observation and reviews.

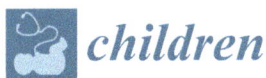

Editorial

Child Injury Prevention: It Is Time to Address the Determinants of Health

Amy E. Peden [1,2,*] and Richard C. Franklin [2]

1. School of Population Health, Faculty of Medicine, University of New South Wales, Kensington, NSW 2052, Australia
2. College of Public Health, Medical and Veterinary Sciences, James Cook University, Townsville, QLD 4811, Australia; richard.franklin@jcu.edu.au
* Correspondence: a.peden@unsw.edu.au

Received: 7 January 2021; Accepted: 13 January 2021; Published: 14 January 2021

Injuries, although almost entirely preventable, accounted for more than 4.4 million deaths and resulted in over 520 million cases of nonfatal injury-related harm globally in 2017 [1]. Road traffic injuries, falls and drowning are leading injury mechanisms [2–4]. However, some population groups are more vulnerable to being injured than others. This Special Issue sought to unpack this concept by exploring the determinants of health and their impact on child injuries.

The determinants of health are a wide group of underlying causes, often referred to as the "causes of the causes" [5], which impact health and wellbeing. Determinants of health include level of education, family income, housing conditions, and the geographical location of place of residence [6]. While it is clear that determinants of health impact wellbeing and quality of life [7–9], more work needs to be done to explore their impact on injury risk. Even more important is the need to identify and quantify the bi-directional benefit of preventing injury and addressing determinants of health [10,11]. This is of importance across all ages; however, the greatest health gains can be made among children and adolescents [12]; hence the focus of this Special Issue.

There are many examples of how determinants of health impact injury risk. These include geographical location, income level and employment. Geographical location impacts availability of medical services, with rural people often located at a larger distance from emergency services, which impacts response times [13]. There are also persistent healthcare workforce shortages [14] resulting in reduced access to services such as occupational therapy for in-home modifications or physiotherapy to help with strength, balance and posture to prevent falls [15].

Similarly, income level impacts injury risk with higher rates of road traffic injuries seen in lower income areas due to differences in roadway design [16]. A low-income household was found to be the single most important predictor for severe paediatric intentional and unintentional injury [17]. Higher rates of fire-related injuries [18] and hot water-related burns and scalds [19] were seen in low-income households, in part due to lower use of protective devices such as smoke alarms and hot water system modifications.

Income level is linked to employment. Research indicates higher rates of suicide [20] and intentional injury [21] among those who are unemployed and higher rates of injury-related fatalities among children in households where no adults are employed [22]. Unemployment is also linked to alcohol and drug abuse [23], another risk factor for a myriad of injury mechanisms.

Education, another determinant of health, is used to impact injury prevention with schools used to deliver messages and information often provided in written form to parents and caregivers to help inform about child and household safety. For example, programs in Australia, Israel and India use the school system to deliver swimming lessons to reduce drowning risk [24], road safety education [25] and fire safety [26].

This Special Issue comprises ten eclectic papers, spanning high income and low- and middle-income contexts, each of which provides a small window into childhood injuries and highlights the need to consider the determinants of health. Common themes to emerge included the impact of socio-economic status on increased child injury risk across a range of injury mechanisms [27–30]. The issue of mobile device use leading to distraction from supervision of children at playgrounds is ubiquitous across high, middle, and low socio-economic areas in developed nations, and leads to increased injury risk [31].

Race, ethnicity and culture were common determinants across several papers, with race and ethnicity being identified as risk factors for work-related fatalities in New Zealand [32], oral self-harm among institutionalized children in Romania [33] and among factors increasing drowning risk [29]. Cultural-related barriers were identified as posing a challenge to the implementation of accepted child drowning prevention interventions in the Sundarbans region of India [30]. Similarly, rurality was found to increase child injury risk in Australia [28] and the Sundarbans region [30].

More broadly, age- and sex-related factors were identified as impacting injury risk during sports and other physical activities, particularly during adolescence [34–36], a period of much physical change.

We encourage our readers to explore these 10 papers and consider the role that determinants of health play in injury risk in their own context. Determinants of health are important, and it is vital to understand how they impact injury, as addressing them will have the additional benefit of reducing injuries. While it may not always be easy it is clear that more work needs to be undertaken around injury and determinants of health. We must ensure that geography, income level, race and ethnicity and education are not barriers to ensuring safety.

Author Contributions: Conceptualization, A.E.P. and R.C.F.; writing—original draft preparation, A.E.P.; writing—review and editing, A.E.P. and R.C.F. All authors have read and agreed to the published version for the manuscript.

Funding: This research received no external funding.

Conflicts of Interest: The authors declare no conflict of interest.

References

1. James, S.L.; Castle, C.D.; Dingels, Z.V.; Fox, J.T.; Hamilton, E.B.; Liu, Z.; Roberts, N.L.S.; Sylte, D.O.; Henry, N.J.; LeGrand, K.E.; et al. Global injury morbidity and mortality from 1990 to 2017: Results from the Global Burden of Disease Study 2017. *Injury Prev.* **2020**, *26* (Suppl. 1), i96–i114. [CrossRef] [PubMed]
2. James, S.L.; Lucchesi, L.R.; Bisignano, C.; Castle, C.D.; Dingels, Z.V.; Fox, J.T.; Hamilton, E.B.; Henry, N.J.; Krohn, K.J.; Liu, Z.; et al. The global burden of falls: Global, regional and national estimates of morbidity and mortality from the Global Burden of Disease Study 2017. *Injury Prev.* **2020**, *26* (Suppl. 1), i3–i11. [CrossRef]
3. James, S.L.; Lucchesi, L.R.; Bisignano, C.; Castle, C.D.; Dingels, Z.V.; Fox, J.T.; Hamilton, E.B.; Liu, Z.; McCracken, D.; Nixon, M.R.; et al. Morbidity and mortality from road injuries: Results from the Global Burden of Disease Study 2017. *Injury Prev.* **2020**, *26* (Suppl. 1), i46–i56. [CrossRef]
4. Franklin, R.C.; Peden, A.E.; Hamilton, E.B.; Bisignano, C.; Castle, C.D.; Dingels, Z.V.; Hay, S.I.; Liu, Z.; Mokdad, A.H.; Roberts, N.L.S.; et al. The burden of unintentional drowning: Global, regional and national estimates of mortality from the Global Burden of Disease 2017 Study. *Injury Prev.* **2020**, *26* (Suppl. 1), i83–i95. [CrossRef] [PubMed]
5. Braveman, P.; Gottlieb, L. The Social Determinants of Health: It's Time to Consider the Causes of the Causes. *Public Health Rep.* **2014**, *129* (Suppl. 2), 19–31. [CrossRef] [PubMed]
6. Marmot, M.; Friel, S.; Bell, R.; Houweling, T.A.J.; Taylor, S. Commission on Social Determinants of Health. *Closing the gap in a generation: Health equity through action on the social determinants of health. Lancet* **2008**, *372*, 1661–1669.
7. Marmot, M. Social determinants of health: From observation to policy. *Med. J. Aust.* **2000**, *172*, 379–382. [CrossRef]

8. Williams, G.H. The determinants of health: Structure, context and agency. *Sociol. Health Illn.* **2003**, *25*, 131–154. [CrossRef]
9. Von Rueden, U.; Gosch, A.; Rajmil, L.; Bisegger, C.; Ravens-Sieberer, U.; the European KIDSCREEN Group. Socioeconomic determinants of health related quality of life in childhood and adolescence: Results from a European study. *J. Epidemiol. Community Health* **2006**, *60*, 130–135.
10. Laflamme, L. Explaining socio-economic differences in injury risks. *Inj. Control Saf. Promot.* **2001**, *8*, 149–153. [CrossRef]
11. Pickett, W.; Molcho, M.; Simpson, K.; Janssen, I.; Kuntsche, E.; Mazur, J.; Harel, Y.; Boyce, W.F. Cross national study of injury and social determinants in adolescents. *Injury Prev.* **2005**, *11*, 213–218. [CrossRef] [PubMed]
12. Harvey, A. Injury prevention and the attainment of child and adolescent health. *Bull. World Health Organ.* **2009**, *87*, 390–394. [CrossRef] [PubMed]
13. Taylor, D.H.; Peden, A.E.; Franklin, R.C. Next steps for drowning prevention in rural and remote Australia: A systematic review of the literature. *Aust. J. Rural Health* **2020**, *28*, 530–542. [CrossRef] [PubMed]
14. Smith, K.B.; Humphreys, J.S.; Wilson, M.G.A. Addressing the health disadvantage of rural populations: How does epidemiological evidence inform rural health policies and research? *Aust. J. Rural. Health* **2008**, *16*, 56–66. [CrossRef]
15. Pighills, A.; Tynan, A.; Furness, L.; Rawle, M. Occupational therapist led environmental assessment and modification to prevent falls: Review of current practice in an Australian rural health service. *Aust. Occup. Ther. J.* **2019**, *66*, 347–361. [CrossRef]
16. Morency, P.; Gauvin, L.; Plante, C.; Fournier, M.; Morency, C. Neighborhood Social Inequalities in Road Traffic Injuries: The Influence of Traffic Volume and Road Design. *Am. J. Public Health* **2012**, *102*, 1112–1119. [CrossRef]
17. Durkin, M.S.; Davidson, L.L.; Kuhn, L.; O'Connor, P.; Barlow, B. Low-income neighborhoods and the risk of severe pediatric injury: A small-area analysis in northern Manhattan. *Am. J. Public Health* **1994**, *84*, 587–592. [CrossRef]
18. Shai, D. Income, Housing, and Fire Injuries: A Census Tract Analysis. *Public Health Rep.* **2006**, *121*, 149–154. [CrossRef]
19. Gielen, A.C.; Shields, W.; McDonald, E.; Frattaroli, S.; Bishai, D.; Ma, X. Home Safety and Low-Income Urban Housing Quality. *Pediatrics* **2012**, *130*, 1053–1059. [CrossRef]
20. Milner, A.J.; Page, A.; Lamontagne, A.D. Duration of unemployment and suicide in Australia over the period 1985–2006: An ecological investigation by sex and age during rising versus declining national unemployment rates. *J. Epidemiol. Community Health* **2013**, *67*, 237–244. [CrossRef]
21. Goins, W.A.; Thompson, J.; Simpkins, C. Recurrent intentional injury. *J. Natl. Med. Assoc.* **1992**, *84*, 431–435. [PubMed]
22. Edwards, P.; Roberts, I.; Green, J.; Lutchmun, S. Deaths from injury in children and employment status in family: Analysis of trends in class specific death rates. *BMJ* **2006**, *333*, 119. [CrossRef] [PubMed]
23. Henkel, D. Unemployment and Substance Use: A Review of the Literature (1990–2010). *Current Drug Abuse Rev.* **2011**, *4*, 4–27. [CrossRef] [PubMed]
24. Franklin, R.; Peden, A.E.; Hodges, S.; Lloyd, N.; Larsen, P.; O'Connor, C.; Scarr, J. Learning to Swim—What influences success? *Int. J. Aquat. Res. Educ.* **2015**, *9*, 220–240. [CrossRef]
25. Ben-Bassat, T.; Avnieli, S. The effect of a road safety educational program for kindergarten children on their parents' behavior and knowledge. *Accid. Anal. Prev.* **2016**, *95*, 78–85. [CrossRef] [PubMed]
26. Moses Rathnakumar, S.P.L.L. The Effectiveness of Video Assisted Teaching on Fire Safety among School Children at Selected School, Kanchipuram District, Tamilnadu. *Med. Leg. Update* **2020**, *20*, 138–140.
27. Guevarra, J.; Peden, A.E.; Orbillo, L.L.; Uy, M.R.S.Z.; Madrilejos, J.J.R.; Go, J.J.L.; Martinez, R.E.C.; Cavinta, L.L.; Franklin, R.C. Preventing Child Drowning in the Philippines: The Need to Address the Determinants of Health. *Children* **2021**, *8*, 29. [CrossRef]
28. Peden, A.; Franklin, R.C. Exploring the Impact of Remoteness and Socio-Economic Status on Child and Adolescent Injury-Related Mortality in Australia. *Children* **2021**, *8*, 5. [CrossRef]
29. Sakamoto, I.; Stempski, S.; Srinivasan, V.; Le, T.; Bennett, E.; Quan, L. Adolescent Water Safety Behaviors, Skills, Training and Their Association with Risk-Taking Behaviors and Risk and Protective Factors. *Children* **2020**, *7*, 301. [CrossRef]

30. Gupta, M.; Roy, S.; Panda, R.; Konwar, P.; Jagnoor, J. Interventions for Child Drowning Reduction in the Indian Sundarbans: Perspectives from the Ground. *Children* **2020**, *7*, 291. [CrossRef]
31. Bury, K.; Jancey, J.; Leavy, J.E. Parent Mobile Phone Use in Playgrounds: A Paradox of Convenience. *Children* **2020**, *7*, 284. [CrossRef] [PubMed]
32. Lilley, R.; McNoe, B.; Davie, G.; de Graaf, B.; Driscoll, T. Work-Related Fatalities Involving Children in New Zealand, 1999–2014. *Children* **2021**, *8*, 4. [CrossRef] [PubMed]
33. Stoica, A.M.S.; Stoica, O.E.; Vlad, R.E.; Pop, A.M.; Monea, M. The Correlation between Oral Self-Harm and Ethnicity in Institutionalized Children. *Children* **2021**, *8*, 2. [CrossRef] [PubMed]
34. Saeki, J.; Iizuka, S.; Sekino, H.; Suzuki, A.; Maemichi, T.; Torii, S. Optimum Angle of Force Production Temporarily Changes Due to Growth in Male Adolescence. *Children* **2021**, *8*, 20. [CrossRef] [PubMed]
35. Karuc, J.; Jelčić, M.; Sorić, M.; Mišigoj-Duraković, M.; Marković, G. Does Sex Dimorphism Exist in Dysfunctional Movement Patterns during the Sensitive Period of Adolescence? *Children* **2020**, *7*, 308. [CrossRef]
36. Sekulic, D.; Prus, D.; Zevrnja, A.; Peric, M.; Zaletel, P. Predicting Injury Status in Adolescent Dancers Involved in Different Dance Styles: A Prospective Study. *Children* **2020**, *7*, 297. [CrossRef]

Publisher's Note: MDPI stays neutral with regard to jurisdictional claims in published maps and institutional affiliations.

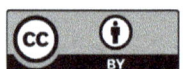

© 2021 by the authors. Licensee MDPI, Basel, Switzerland. This article is an open access article distributed under the terms and conditions of the Creative Commons Attribution (CC BY) license (http://creativecommons.org/licenses/by/4.0/).

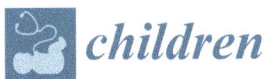

Article

Interventions for Child Drowning Reduction in the Indian Sundarbans: Perspectives from the Ground

Medhavi Gupta [1], Sujoy Roy [2], Ranjan Panda [2], Pompy Konwar [3] and Jagnoor Jagnoor [3,*]

1. The George Institute for Global Health Australia, University of New South Wales, Level 5, 1 King St, Newtown, NSW 2042, Australia; mgupta@georgeinstitute.org.au
2. Child in Need Institute, Daulatpur, Pailan, South 24 Parganas, West Bengal 700104, India; sujoy@cinindia.org (S.R.); ranjan@cinindia.org (R.P.)
3. Injury Division, The George Institute for Global Health India, 311-312, Third Floor, Elegance Tower, Plot No. 8, Jasola District Centre, New Delhi 110025, India; pkonwar@georgeinstitute.org.in
* Correspondence: jjagnoor1@georgeinstitute.org.in; Tel.: +91-11-4158-8091-93

Received: 23 October 2020; Accepted: 11 December 2020; Published: 14 December 2020

Abstract: Drowning is a leading cause of child death in the coastal Sundarbans region of India due to the presence of open water, lack of supervision and poor infrastructure, but no prevention programs are currently implemented. The World Health Organization has identified interventions that may prevent child drowning in rural low-and middle-income country contexts, including the provision of home-based barriers, supervised childcare, swim and rescue training and first responder training. Child health programs should consider the local context and identify barriers for implementation. To ensure the sustainability of any drowning prevention programs implemented, we conducted a qualitative study to identify the considerations for the implementation of these interventions, and to understand how existing government programs could be leveraged. We also identified key stakeholders for involvement. We found that contextual factors such as geography, cultural beliefs around drowning, as well as skillsets of local people, would influence program delivery. Government programs such as accredited social health activists (ASHAs) and self-help groups could be leveraged for program implementation, while Anganwadi centres would require additional support due to poor resourcing. Gaining government permissions to change Anganwadi processes to provide childcare services may be challenging. The results showed that adapting drowning programs to the Sundarbans context presents unique challenges and program customisation.

Keywords: drowning; child health; injury; low-and middle-income country; India; preventative medicine; implementation science; qualitative research

1. Introduction

Drowning is a leading cause of morbidity and mortality in low-and middle-income countries (LMICs) [1]. Of these deaths, 62,000 occur in India, where drowning is the foremost cause of death by injury for children aged 1–4 years [2]. Rural and remote coastal regions in LMICs present the highest risk of child drowning. Rural, forested Sundarbans region in the northern state of West Bengal is one such area. Sundarbans experiences frequent flooding, a presence of open water, poor infrastructure and poor health systems [3–5]. A recent survey in the Sundarbans found particularly high rates of drowning in children aged 1–9 years where it is likely the leading cause of death in this group [6].

The World Health Organization (WHO, Geneva, Switzerland) recommends the implementation of four effective community-based interventions in rural LMIC settings to reduce drowning in young children. These interventions are activities that may be feasibly implemented in low-resource contexts and have been shown to reduce drowning burden [1]. These interventions are: the installation of home-based barriers controlling access to water (such as playpens and door barriers), the provision of supervised safe spaces with capable child care, teaching school-aged children basic swimming and rescue skills and training adult bystanders in rescue and resuscitation [1]. Previous research has shown that communities in the Sundarbans consider drowning a health issue [7]. Despite this perception and the high rates of drowning, there are no preventive measures implemented in the region.

Previous research and experience in the sustainable program design has shown that it is essential to understand the context, local perceptions and possible implementation-related challenges before designing and implementing community-based programs [8–10]. The identification of key stakeholders that may support or inhibit implementation must also be identified [11,12]. These stakeholders can include members of the community who can influence program engagement, as well as governmental or organisational leaders whose support and buy in is beneficial for community acceptance and access to local resources.

A key strategy that improves program sustainability is linking program goals with government priorities and leveraging existing programs [13,14]. A comprehensive policy review of West Bengal and National policy found three government programs that may be appropriate to build upon to implement drowning reduction programs: the integrated child development scheme (ICDS), self-help group (SHGs) schemes and the accredited social health activist (ASHA) program [15]. The federal ICDS program was introduced in 1975 and aims to provide free childcare services to children aged 3–6 years through village-based Anganwadi centres [16]. The implementation and reach of these centres are highly variable across the Sundarbans, and many centres do not provide the childcare services promised in the policy (Biswas and Chattapadhyay, 2001; Biswas et al., 2010). The quality improvement of the ICDS program has the potential to provide structured supervision, for injury prevention. The SHG scheme aims to reduce rural poverty and increase household income through the setup of self-help groups in villages, primarily with women. Some SHGs also become involved in community projects, such as the provision of midday meals in schools [17]. ASHA workers are community-based health workers who focus on child and maternal health on an incentive-based system, and have close ties with mothers [18,19]. Both SHGs and ASHAs may be leveraged in the provision of community-education such as rescue and resuscitation training and supporting families in building and maintaining home-based barriers.

We conducted the formative contextual analysis required to design a sustainable drowning reduction program for the Sundarbans, as guided by WHO recommendations. The objectives were as follows: (1) identify community perceptions and preferences towards the recommended drowning interventions; (2) explore the feasibility of leveraging ICDS, ASHA or SHG programs for the delivery of drowning reduction interventions; (3) identify contextual challenges and considerations for the design and delivery of the program; and (4) identify key stakeholders who should be engaged during the development and implementation of the program.

2. Materials and Methods

We applied qualitative methods to understand the micro context in which drowning reduction interventions could be delivered in the Sundarbans. In-depth interviews (IDIs), focus group discussions (FGDs) and observations were conducted and triangulated to develop this understanding. IDIs gave insights into individual-level perspectives, and FGDs were used to identify community norms and perceptions. Observations allowed for the better understanding of government program operations and systems. Qualitative methodology was guided by the Consolidated Criteria for Reporting Qualitative Research (COREQ) (see Supplementary Table S1) [20].

2.1. Data Collection

Data collection was conducted in partnership with a local non-governmental organization (NGO), the Child in Need Institute (CINI). CINI has operated child and maternal health programs in rural West

Bengal for the past 46 years and has extensive connections with communities and local government in the Sundarbans region. The data collection of community-based participants was completed by two male data collectors recruited by CINI, managed by S.R. and R.P. who work as the programs' manager and director, respectively. The data collectors had previous experience in qualitative research in West Bengal and were trained by the researchers in the study aims and tools. One of the data collectors had experience conducting qualitative data collection in the Sundarbans and was familiar with the community. M.G. conducted English-language interviews, such as with grassroots organisations.

All data collection occurred face-to-face. IDIs and FGDs were held in locations that best suited participants, such as in community schools or Anganwadi centres. In addition to the data collectors and participants, NGO partner facilitators were present for some IDIs, FGDs and observations to lend logistical support. All IDIs and FGDs were audio recorded and lasted between 30 and 90 min. Field notes were also taken by one data collector and collated to make key point summaries of each IDI, FGD and observation on a daily basis, which was shared with the research team.

All Bengali transcripts were translated into English for analysis. No interviews were repeated. Transcripts were not returned to participants for comment due to the logistical and literacy barriers.

2.2. Participants

All participants were adults over the age of 18. A minimum of three IDIs and two FGDs were conducted for each stakeholder type to ensure the capture of varying responses. Stakeholder types interviewed included (1) community-level participants including men, women and leaders, (2) government program participants and delivery staff, and (3) grassroots organisations. These stakeholder types are described in detail below. This range of stakeholders enabled for the identification of contextual considerations from the perspectives of program implementers and beneficiaries and ensured that individuals from different levels of the social hierarchy were heard. Data collection ceased once saturation in each type was reached.

2.2.1. Community-Level Participants

Community men, women and leader participants were recruited through convenience sampling. The partner NGO first approached local government bodies for permission to conduct the interviews. Data collectors then entered the communities as recommended by the Gram Panchayats (who are the lowest local government body representing a group of villages) and engaged local leaders such as ASHA and Anganwadi workers, who introduced the data collectors to possible participants. Participants were required to be parents and usual residents of the community living there for the past three years. Participants were recruited across all 19 blocks of the Sundarbans to ensure a range of perspectives.

These participants provided insights into community acceptance and perceptions towards drowning interventions, as well as possible barriers and enablers to implementation in the local context. A total of ten IDIs and nine FGDs were conducted with community-level participants, with men and women equally represented.

2.2.2. Government Program Participants

Anganwadi workers, SHG members and ASHA workers were approached through purposive sampling after entering communities in which permission for data collection had been granted by local government officials. Communities had one or two ASHA and Anganwadi workers each, so whoever was available upon contact was scheduled for interview. As self-help group members were found in many households, community members would lead data collectors to the closest home of a member. These participants were included if they were active in their respective programs for a minimum of 6 months within the Sundarbans region.

Observations of SHG meetings and Anganwadi centres were conducted to understand their operations. By policy, one Anganwadi centre is required to serve a population of 1000 people, providing any children aged 3–6 years old with early childhood education activities for two hours each day along with a nutritious meal. Each centre should have one Anganwadi worker and one helper, and usually operates between 7 and 10 a.m. We observed the children who came to the Anganwadi Centres and provided insights into how children interacted with the Anganwadi workers, as well as the ground realities of the program delivery. Observations of SHGs identified decision-making methods and revealed the role of SHGs in the community. Anganwadi centres and SHGs for observations were purposively selected in partnership with a local NGO working with these programmes to cover a range of performance levels. Nine government program participants (ASHA workers, Anganwadi workers and SHG members) were interviewed. Two FGDs with SHG members were also held and three observations each were conducted at Anganwadi centres and SHG meetings.

2.2.3. Grassroots Organisations

Interviews were conducted with the individuals from organisations working in the child health, education, safety or nutrition in the Sundarbans or other similar rural contexts in West Bengal. This provided insights into the considerations and challenges related to delivering grassroots programs in the Sundarbans. Potential participants were introduced to the researchers by our partner NGO and were required to have oversight over program delivery for at least one year. Three representatives from grassroots organisations were interviewed.

2.3. Tools and Transcriptions

Tools for all IDIs, FGDs and Observations were developed before the commencement of data collection and translated into Bengali. The data collection guides were semi- structured to ensure all domains relevant to research questions were covered.

All participants were also shown a pictorial presenting the WHO-recommended drowning interventions. Barriers were described as any physical object preventing children's access to water such as playpens, door barriers or fencing. Childcare was described as any group-based supervision in an enclosed space. Swimming lessons encompassed both swim and rescue training skills, and first responder training was described as training adults on how to save children if they fall into water or start drowning.

2.4. Ethics

All participants provided verbal or written informed consent depending on their literacy level. Ethical approval was granted by the University of New South Wales Human Research Ethics Committee (HC 190274) in Sydney, Australia and The George Institute for Global Health (India) Ethics Committee (06/2019) in New Dealhi, India.

2.5. Analysis

Analysis of the transcripts was completed using NVivo 12 [21]. Narrative analysis was used where key themes under each of the broad research objectives were derived. All transcripts were coded against a priori key themes based on the research questions, including the acceptability of each of the WHO drowning reduction programs, and considerations for the implementation and feasibility of using government programs to deliver the programs. Subsequent sub-themes were developed under each of these based on commonalities and diversified perspectives from participants. We also triangulated different sources of data by coding for the type of stakeholder and type of qualitative method (IDI, FGD, observation) to assess congruent and different perspectives across genders and participant type as well as to compare individual and community-level viewpoints [22]. The two independent reviewers (M.G. and P.K.) discussed their results and discrepancies before finalising the key findings.

Stakeholders were identified and then allocated to level of power and interest as based on Mendelow's Matrix [23]. The level of power describes the stakeholder's influence over program success, and the level of interest reflects the impacts of the program on the stakeholder. The framework was used to identify the correct engagement strategies for each of the stakeholders based on their framework allocation.

3. Results

Refusal to participate in the study was less than 10%. Below we discuss the overall and intervention-specific considerations for program implementation in the Sundarbans, the feasibility of using government programs and identify the stakeholders who must be involved in program design and delivery.

The Supplementary File (Table S2 in Supplementary File S2) depicts illustrative quotes from the following analysis. Figure 1 below provides a summary of the main enablers and barriers identified for the intervention implementation, from the perspective of program beneficiaries (demand-side) and from the perspective of program implementers (supply-side).

	Demand-side considerations	Supply-side considerations
Enablers	• Acceptability and appetite for interventions • Low levels of religious or caste-based discrimination	• Regular community engagement • Well connected and willing ASHAs* and SHG** members, with permissions to engage easily attainable
Barriers	• Affordability • Belief children can swim • Poor suitability of public ponds • Cultural beliefs on appropriate rescue behaviours	• Lack of skills and resources • Requirement for customisable home-based barriers • Poor Anganwadi centre conditions and burdening of workers, and difficultly in gaining permissions to engage program • Poor geographic connectivity

* Accredited Social Health Activists
** Self-help group

Figure 1. Key contextual enablers and barriers to implementation identified by participants.

3.1. Considerations for Program Design and Delivery

A range of considerations were identified that applied to all drowning reduction interventions.

3.1.1. Acceptability across All Interventions

Participants showed heterogeneity in preferences between the interventions. All interventions were generally considered acceptable. Some participants recognised that each of the interventions targeted different age groups and expressed a need for an age-targeted and comprehensive approach (Refs 1 and 2 in Table S2 of Supplementary File S2).

3.1.2. Affordability

Cost to households was a concern for all interventions. Many participants stated that with limited resources and competing priorities, a drowning reduction intervention would not be affordable for households. The home-based barriers' intervention was considered the most feasible for self-funding as it was viewed as a one-time investment, with maintenance being of negligible cost. They also noted that parents who are unable to afford services may cause problems and complain if excluded.

Some participants suggested that families could pay different amounts depending on their income level, which could be pooled together to fund the program (Ref 3 in Table S2).

3.1.3. Community Engagement and Ownership

Consistent community engagement through regular meetings, showcases, theatre and household visits were identified as important to implementation success. Participants noted that program ownership should be transferred to the community over time, such as by setting up an implementation committee. Participants noted that without consistent engagement, people may fall back into previous habits and stop engaging with the program (Refs 4 and 5 in Table S2).

Community leaders and grassroots organisations' participants also discussed the importance of regular program monitoring. They stressed that communities and implementing agencies should work in partnership to ensure that interventions were being implemented and used as designed (Ref 6 in Table S2).

3.1.4. Resources and Skill Set

Participants also noted that geographical and infrastructure barriers such as the road quality and the connectivity of many areas were challenges. Participants suggested that local resources should be used where possible, such as bamboo from the area for barriers (Ref 7 in Table S2).

Grassroots organisations also noted that finding capable human resources was often challenging due to lower educational attainment in the region and the migration of skilled workers to the cities. Benefits and incentives would need to meet community expectations to recruit capable staff. However, the programs would provide an opportunity for women to access employment, as few jobs were available to them post high-school. Program providers may also face risks if a child was injured under their care from angry parents (Ref 8 in Table S2).

3.1.5. Social Class

Participants largely stated that caste and religion did not present an issue. Community member participants did not anticipate any discrimination towards potential intervention beneficiaries. However, some instances of discrimination against Muslim Anganwadi workers by Hindus, or against Hindu SHG members by Muslims, were reported by government program participants during IDIs. Government program participants also stated that political party affiliation may affect cooperation and participation in interventions. Program staff from different political parties may refuse to work together or may discriminate against communities from other parties (Refs 9 and 10 in Table S2).

Some participants also noted that as Muslims were relatively economically disadvantaged and conservative, they may have less capacity or willingness to pay (Ref 11 in Table S2).

3.2. Intervention-Specific Considerations

In addition to findings to guide general program implementation, specific considerations were identified for each of the WHO-recommended drowning interventions.

3.2.1. Home-Based Barriers

Home-based barriers were largely acceptable to communities provided certain conditions were met. Many adults noted that this method was used previously in their childhood but concerns for children's mental wellbeing stopped the practice as a lack of movement and social interaction with other children was considered detrimental. The intervention was also only considered suitable for younger children under the age of 2–2.5 years, as older children would try to climb the barriers (Ref 12 in Table S2).

The feasibility of different types of barriers varied between households. Some participants noted that families may struggle to keep door barriers and pond fencing gates closed due to regular access. Building and maintaining fencing around all ponds within 20–50 m of homes may not be feasible due to the large number of ponds in some villages. Some community members expressed concerns over restricting children's movement in playpens which may be detrimental to their development (Refs 13 and 14 in Table S2).

For playpens, many participants noted that an adult would still need to be present to ensure safety. Participants also suggested that door barriers or fencing gates could be made lower so that adults could climb over without opening them, increasing convenience and reducing the likelihood of it being left open. One participant suggested that young children from nearby homes could be kept together in a large playpen in the middle of the homes with one adult supervising (Refs 15 and 16 in Table S2).

Some participants identified that locally trained professionals were required to build and install the barriers to maintain quality (Ref 17 in Table S2).

3.2.2. Childcare and Supervision-Based Programs

Childcare was largely acceptable in communities, especially as it provided parents with relief from supervision while they worked and offered an opportunity for children to participate in early childhood education, including for children with disabilities who often had few avenues for learning (Ref 18 in Table S2).

However, some participants were concerned for children's safety, as one adult was not considered enough supervision for a group. The region had also experienced instances of child trafficking. Parents were also busy during the day and often restricted in their ability to pick up and drop off children. This issue would be exacerbated in monsoon season when roads are flooded. Parents were also concerned that young children below the age of two years old would not engage with activities and experience separation anxiety.

Participants offered a range of suggestions for childcare implementation. Children could be divided into groups by age so they could be engaged in age-appropriate activities (Refs 19 and 20 in Table S2).

Participants stated that more than one carer was required to look after children to ensure they remained supervised if one child had to be taken for a bathroom break. They also supported the employment of a trusted and known local woman with training for the role (Ref 21 in Table S2).

The provision of toys, activities and learning material was also required to ensure that parents and children would be interested. A gated 'community playground' was suggested to provide an outdoor play space. Pick up and drop off services would increase attendance. Toilet and water facilities were also required. Food provision would improve attendance as both parents and children would be more satisfied. The venue was also required to be large and secure for safe play (Refs 22 and 23 in Table S2).

The preferred hours for the childcare services varied. Many participants, especially mothers, noted that parents were busy in both the morning and afternoon but were home for lunch. They suggested a session both before and after lunch (Ref 24 in Table S2).

3.2.3. Swim and Rescue Training

Many participants believed that children had adequate swimming skills from informal lessons provided by parents in family ponds but were interested in rescue training. Participants acknowledged that some individuals did not have access to a pond to learn or did not have time to teach their children swimming, so classes were important for them. Children would also be motivated by the chance to participate in regional swimming competitions (Ref 25 in Table S2).

Ponds in this region are mostly privately owned and used for washing, cleaning and fishing. Some participants reported that there were no common ponds large enough for training in their communities, so private ponds were required. Seeking someone who would lend their pond may be difficult. In addition, many ponds were unsuitable, being dirty and deep (Ref 26 in Table S2).

For quality control, participants suggested that guidelines for pond selection should be developed, covering location, cleanliness and depth criteria. Safety and rescue material should also be available, and platforms built for access to the pond. A changing room would also reduce community push-back as children would not travel home in wet clothing (Refs 27 and 28 in Table S2).

Some participants believed a trainer from outside the community would be better respected by the community, while others preferred a local who would have better relationships with the community and would be more consistently available (Refs 29 and 30 in Table S2).

3.2.4. First Responder Program

The first responder training was acceptable to most participants, especially parents of young children as they were interested in learning how to protect them (Ref 31 in Table S2).

However, cultural beliefs may remain a barrier to appropriate responses. During drowning events, people in the communities had previously ignored health advice from community health workers such as ASHAs and conducted traditional responses, such as calling a local village doctor or performing rituals on the water. These responses had led to delays in children receiving appropriate medical care (Ref 32 in Table S2).

3.2.5. Indigenous Interventions for Child Safety

A range of other intervention ideas and solutions were offered by participants. Many stated that awareness programs were required in parallel to drowning interventions to educate communities about the risks of drowning and ensure sustained behaviour change. Awareness activities would also seek to dispel harmful beliefs about drowning, such as on cultural post-drowning rituals that led to delays in children receiving first aid. Participants noted that other existing programs in communities with established activities, such as vaccination programs, could be leveraged for awareness activities (Ref 33 in Table S2).

Native interventions employed by communities were also identified. Some parents tied their children to their waist or to the house with rope while they worked. Others kept their children locked inside the home alone when they were away (Ref 34 in Table S2).

Other possible solutions were offered such as providing vans for school children or organising 'walking buses' where children would travel to school together, and teaching children to have a 'shore guard' during play time where one child kept watch from the pond's edge.

3.3. Use of Government Programs in Drowning Intervention Delivery

Possible roles in the implementation of drowning interventions were identified for existing government programs in communities.

3.3.1. ASHA Workers

ASHA workers were interested in supporting the dissemination of drowning reduction programs and were considered suitable for providing training due to their reputation as health workers. ASHA workers were already regularly visiting mothers and children up to the age of 5 years old and could encourage the use of drowning interventions and conduct checks of home-based barriers. However, some participants noted that not all ASHA workers had strong relationships with communities, where their health communications such as community meetings were now largely ignored due to fatigue with repeated advice and instructions (Ref 35 in Table S2).

ASHAs already had some skills in rescue and response. Some ASHAs expressed a desire to learn first aid more comprehensively to perform better in their roles. They were also willing to train others in their communities. However, ASHA workers stated that their work was highly unpredictable as they often responded to calls of women in labour, and so could not provide training and childcare for large blocks of time (Ref 36 in Table S2).

ASHA workers worked on an incentive-based system and expected added payment for services. (Ref 37 in Table S2).

3.3.2. Self-Help Groups

Self-help group (SHG) members were primarily interested in the delivery of childcare services and suggested they may provide pick up and drop off services for children to and from swimming and childcare interventions. Some SHGs were already involved in delivering government programs, such as the mid-day meal scheme in schools. They expected to be paid for involvement (Ref 38 in Table S2).

Many households in communities had at least one SHG member, making them well connected. They would be able to support community engagement activities, such as through organising mothers' meetings and household visits (Ref 39 in Table S2).

Some possible barriers for the engagement of SHGs were identified. Firstly, many were busy with their family businesses and may have minimal time to be engaged. Secondly, some were concerned about their lower levels of education and stressed the need for comprehensive training. Lastly, some SHGs others faced challenges with the engagement of all members. The supervision of SHGs also varied and the management of SHGs involved in drowning intervention delivery may require a separate system (Ref 40 in Table S2).

Community leaders and grassroots organisation participants noted that SHG members were easier to engage in drowning interventions than Anganwadi centres or ASHAs as they required fewer government permissions. However, some SHG members may face restriction from their husbands or families due to cultural constraints on women's mobility and employment (Ref 41 in Table S2).

3.3.3. Anganwadi Centres (ICDS Program)

Anganwadi centres were considered possibly suitable for the implementation of childcare supervision and parent engagement activities. Centres were usually open from 7 a.m. to 9 or 10 a.m. with 20–30 children attending each day. Some centres already provided a limited range of childcare activities, and parents left their children for 1–2 h with the Anganwadi centre.

However, there was great variability described and observed in the quality of services. Participants reported that many Anganwadi centres only provided food and no childcare services. This may be due to the lack of an appropriately enclosed venue, lack of training for Anganwadi workers and parents' low trust in the centre. In two out of three of the Anganwadi centre observations, the Anganwadi worker did not facilitate any games or activities. Many participants also complained of a lack of educational materials and repeating activities (Refs 42 and 43 in Table S2).

In addition, many venues lacked toilets and water and children were left alone if a child was taken to relieve themselves. Many participants reported that Anganwadi venues did not have enough space for both cooking and childcare activities and were not safely enclosed. A barrier to finding appropriate venues was that the local government requested private land to be leased for 50–100 years for the centres, which few people agreed to. Parents also did not always have time to pick and drop their children, especially if the centre was at a further distance from their home (Ref 44 in Table S2).

Anganwadi workers were also burdened with their duties and had limited training. Anganwadi workers had other responsibilities such as conducting surveys for the Department of Health on sanitation and maintaining the registers of children. They were often busy until 12 p.m. after the centre closed at 10 a.m. They also struggled to cook, clean and provide childcare activities at once. Many centres did not have an Anganwadi assistant allocated or regularly attending. Anganwadi workers also reported being unsatisfied with the pay (Refs 45 and 46 in Table S2).

Anganwadi workers were trained when they joined the program, but the training did not cover ECE activities in detail. They were provided limited ongoing support, where meetings with Panchayat officials who oversaw the implementation of ICDS, visits from supervisors and block-level offices were infrequent (Ref 47 in Table S2).

Parents also complained that food was of inadequate quantity. Improper food provision meant many parents had lost trust in the Anganwadi centres. Anganwadi workers and community leaders stated that poor food quality was due to resourcing issues such as insufficient money provided for ingredients amidst rising prices and a lack of water and sanitation in the venues (Ref 48 in Table S2).

Making changes to Anganwadi centres at a local level required permissions from both Health and Women and Child Development representatives at the block level. Block-level representatives (the level of government just above Gram Panchayats) are responsible for monitoring program performance. Although Gram Panchayats are responsible for the program implementation of ICDS, they do not have the permission to make operational changes as their targets and delivery requirements are set by State policy and enforced by block-level supervisors. Grassroots organisation and community leader participants noted that engaging block-level representatives may be challenging without higher state-level permissions which may take months to obtain. Grassroot participants had experienced that government departments were cautious about giving permissions when liabilities were not clear. These participants stated that running a parallel program for childcare may be easier than using the ICDS (Refs 49 and 50 in Table S2).

A few communities had parallel NGO-run childcare programs which children attended after visiting the Anganwadi centre. These programs were considered of better quality than Anganwadi centres (Ref 51 in Table S2).

3.3.4. Other Community Programs

Local youth clubs were identified by many participants as potential implementers of programs. These clubs were organisations run by youth and overseen by Gram Panchayats. They aimed to engage young people in self and community development activities (Ref 52 in Table S2).

3.4. Stakeholder Analysis

A range of stakeholders important to program delivery were identified. The placement of these stakeholders along Mendelow's Matrix is presented in Figure 2 below.

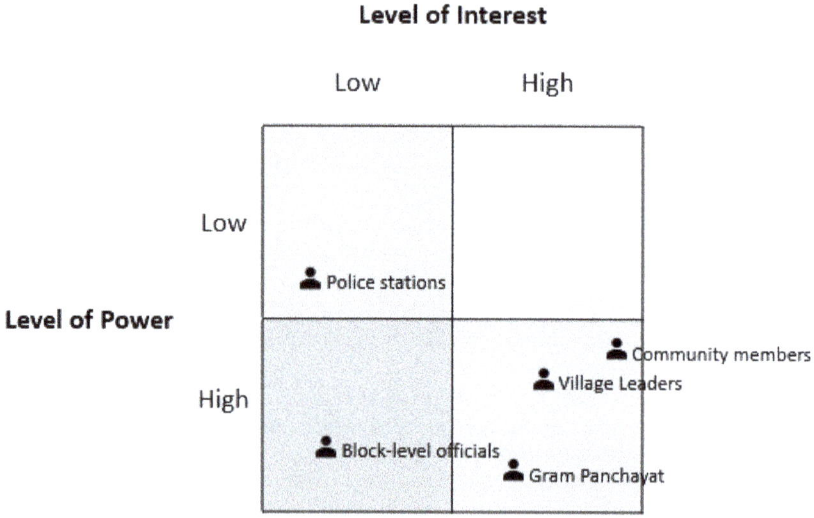

Figure 2. Stakeholder placement in Mendelow's Matrix.

3.4.1. Block-Level Officials

Block-level government officials represent the district-level government at a smaller administration level. Information and gaining permissions from the block-level government would ensure there were no complaints later down the line, especially if existing government programs were used (Ref 53 in Table S2).

3.4.2. Gram Panchayat

The Gram Panchayat was the lowest local government body. They were responsible for the ICDS and SHG programs. They ran awareness and door-to-door campaigns on issues such as dengue. Most participants stated that any implementation activities must involve the Gram Panchayat. The Gram Panchayat would give permission for activities occurring in communities and were influential over village leaders. They could also assist in the recruitment of suitable program staff, the identification of venues for intervention activities and assist in resolving arising challenges. However, Gram Panchayats were unlikely to have their own funding to support the interventions (Ref 54 in Table S2).

Issues with nepotism in the Gram Panchayat operations were reported. Positions and resources were given to family members to run schemes who had limited incentive to ensure quality. This may present a challenge with recruitment. Panchayats were also not always responsive to requests for resources. One Anganwadi worker had been submitting applications for a new venue for two years with no response (Ref 55 in Table S2).

3.4.3. Community Leaders

Many communities had a leader or influential educated individuals. These individuals would need to be engaged before implementation to assist with delivery and community mobilisation. This may include the village head and teachers. They also oversaw the activities of SHGs (Ref 56 in Table S2).

3.4.4. Local Police Stations

Local police stations would become involved if any accidents or issues occurred, so participants suggested that they should be made aware of any intervention activities. This would ensure they were willing to assist if challenges arise (Ref 57 in Table S2).

3.4.5. Community Members

Community members should take an active role in the implementation of the drowning interventions, providing inputs in locations and responsibility. Community-level participants were interested in supporting the programs (Ref 58 in Table S2).

3.4.6. Engagement Strategies

As per the placement on Mendelow's Matrix, community members, village leaders and Gram Panchayats had high levels of power over program implementation and a high level of interest. Hence, these stakeholders should be actively and directly engaged in intervention design, development and implementation. Block-level officials have a high level of power, but lower levels of interest and should be engaged for permission and kept informed.

4. Discussion

Our analysis of micro and community-level stakeholder perceptions towards drowning interventions revealed opportunities for the implementation of drowning reduction programs in the Sundarbans.

The findings suggested that all recommended interventions must be introduced together in a comprehensive program for maximum effectiveness. According to the participants, barrier-based interventions were considered appropriate for 1–2-year-old children, childcare for 3–5-year-old children, and swim and rescue training for children over the age of 6 years. Participants were largely homogenous in this view, given cultural norms around childrearing and care. In addition, first responder training was perceived as important to encourage appropriate post-drowning actions. The age-appropriateness identified by participants for each intervention was in line with WHO implementation guidelines [24].

While the core components of these interventions would remain the same, such as ensuring that childcare spaces are secure and are provided during at-risk hours, the delivery processes of a comprehensive program should be adapted to the Sundarbans context. These changeable program characteristics include the nature of the community delivery agents, the capacity and capability of available workforce, availability of infrastructure and resources, partnership opportunities, methods of communication, and cultural adaptations such as changes to language and messaging [25,26]. The design and development of the comprehensive drowning program should involve community groups and stakeholders to ensure sustainability.

In this study, some specific intervention adaptations were identified as appropriate to the Sundarbans. An essential finding for the barrier-based intervention was that the preferred type of barrier varied by household. Hence, a drowning program may seek to deliver customised barriers for each household. Participants identified that childcare services should have an adequate child to caretaker ratio to ensure child security and provide pick up and drop off services to encourage attendance. These provisions to ensure child safety and support for attendance were also identified in international guidelines on childcare provision [27,28]. Participants were similarly concerned with safety for swim and rescue training services.

Participants also noted the need for complementary awareness activities, such as to dispel improper beliefs around effective child rescue techniques. Common responses to child drowning incidents involve engaging local quack doctors to perform rituals and trying to remove water by spinning the child over an adult's head [7,29]. Changing problematic norms and beliefs is an important step in behaviour change, and Sundarbans communities must be informed that such actions do not save children [30–33]. However, awareness itself is not sufficient to change behaviour, and must be accompanied with the removal of obstacles to change and capacity building [31,34]. Hence, awareness and first responder training in the Sundarbans may also need to target local 'quack' doctors who have some authority over community responses to drowning and may override individuals advocating for the administration of proper first aid. Ensuring that these local doctors themselves promote and administer appropriate first response may be critical for sustainable impact.

The sustainability of programs improves when they leverage existing government structures [9]. Our findings suggest that the ICDS, ASHA and SHG programs may provide platforms through which a drowning reduction program may be promoted and implemented. ASHA workers may play a promotive and monitoring role for the program and may also be involved in first responder training. However, many ASHA workers are overburdened with their duties and their drowning program role may be more sustainable if it is incorporated into their existing activities, such as providing barrier monitoring support as part of their regular household visits [35]. SHG members also showed willingness to be involved with drowning reduction activities and provided a network through which program activities can be advertised. Members were also available to be recruited for program delivery. ASHA worker and SHG members' performance may also vary depending on the frequency of visits from government supervisors, so independent program monitoring may be required [36].

Concerns were raised around the utilisation of Anganwadi centres for childcare services. The ICDS program suffered from unsafe venues, lack of Anganwadi training and poor sanitary conditions. The local government also had limited authority over the changing operations of centres to include more hours of childcare, requiring permissions from state-level bureaucrats, which may take time given decision makers are risk-averse to changes. NGO participants suggested that a parallel program was more feasible. The long-term goal of health program design, implementation and scale up is often the uptake of these programs by government, as this improves the likelihood of sustained funding and delivery [14,37]. A parallel program may be less likely to be picked up by the government as the ICDS program already provides childcare services as per policy. In addition, optimising existing Anganwadi centres may require fewer resources than opening new centres. Community and local-government engagement activities should seek to decide on which model has long-term feasibility: optimising Anganwadi centres or running a parallel program.

Key facilitating factors that will enable implementation were identified by participants. Consistent community engagement and buy in of local leaders were essential. This is well founded in other LMIC contexts [38]. However, participants also noted that local government was affected by nepotistic practices that may affect program quality. In West Bengal, a study found that local government members were allocating agricultural resources to communities with more power, land and connections [39]. Hence, strict protocols and oversight may be required to ensure the equitable distribution of program resources.

Community participants advocated for local individuals to be trained as childcare and swim training providers. Implementation analyses have shown that local community-based workers best operate when they have access to resources, training and monitoring. Additionally, the building of soft skills, such as communication and leadership, is vital [40]. Community worker engagement and management should be carefully defined and involve incentive structures appropriate to the context and matching community expectations [41–43].

Participants also noted that community-level committees are effective mechanisms through which residents can own programs and monitor implementation. These committees can also be engaged in advocacy and engagement activities and be instrumental in ensuring that implementation responds to community needs [26]. Increased community ownership of health programs may lead to better adaptation to the context and a greater likelihood of sustainability and acceptability [12,44]. However, the underlying assumption of all participants was that an NGO with expertise in child programs, such as CINI, would take primary lead in implementing and supporting community-level committees and program delivery. CINI has over 46 years of experience in delivering child programs in rural regions of West Bengal and is a suitable lead agency.

The development of the intervention may also consider the incorporation of other ideas. Although there is limited evidence on the effectiveness (and on the ethics) of tying children indoors to the ends of rope, there is some evidence that walking school bus programs can prevent injury in children [45]. While these have previously been used to reduce road traffic injuries, in the context of the Sundarbans, this may help reduce drowning events during commutes to school [46]. However, this intervention does not target the age group with the largest burden—1–4-year-old children.

To ensure the community ownership and development of an acceptable and feasible program, the next step of program design should involve community participatory approaches [10,47]. The present study found a range of issues that may affect program delivery, such as unpredictable geography, poor connectivity, religion and the caste of program providers, remoteness, poverty, poor government program monitoring structures, requirement for appropriate incentives, recruitment challenges and the availability of appropriate venues. Communities are the best informants for how context-specific issues can be addressed and managed [48]. Participatory approaches will also improve community buy-in and redistribute the power of change into the community's hands [49]. The range of stakeholders as identified in the stakeholder analysis and should be appropriately engaged, starting with Gram Panchayat and block-level officials and moving to individual community leaders and members. No lifesaving organisations were identified which conduct drowning prevention activities, which was unsurprising as lifesaving organisations have had limited contribution to drowning prevention capacity development and advocacy in remote regions of India.

Limitations of This Study

Due to ethical constraints, we were not able to gather information on participants' caste or religion. It is unclear if the perspectives found are representative across a range of religious groups. In addition, some government program workers were recruited with assistance from Gram Panchayats. These may have been the more active and well performing workers and may not be fully representative of typical programs. This was particularly mitigated by ensuring at least one poor performing worker of each type was purposively recruited.

5. Conclusions

The Sundarbans are a high-risk region for child drowning, and we aimed to identify the mechanisms and considerations for the implementation of drowning reduction programs in the region. We found that program design should consider contextual factors such as geography, cultural beliefs around drowning, skillsets of local people and household-level needs. It was found feasible to leverage government programs such as ASHA workers and SHGs for program recruitment and implementation, while the optimisation of Anganwadi centres for the provision of childcare may be challenging due to poor resourcing and permissions required. Community-based young clubs were also possible implementers of programs. Program development and implementation should involve a range of stakeholders such as local government members, block and district-level health and development officials, community leaders and residents. The results show that the development of drowning reduction programs in rural LMIC contexts should be catered to the local social and environmental context to ensure acceptability and feasibility.

Supplementary Materials: The following are available online at http://www.mdpi.com/2227-9067/7/12/291/s1, Table S1: Consolidated criteria for reporting qualitative studies (COREQ): 32-item checklist, Table S2: Illustrative quotations by theme.

Author Contributions: M.G. and J.J. conceptualised and designed the study. M.G. developed the data collection tools with support from J.J., S.R. and R.P. S.R. and R.P. coordinated and supervised data collection and quality maintenance activities. M.G. and P.K. carried out the analysis. M.G. drafted the manuscript with inputs from P.K. and J.J. All authors have read and agreed to the published version of the manuscript.

Funding: This project was supported by the University of New South Wales through the Research Training Program Scholarship (awarded to M.G., no award number) and National Health and Medical Research Council (Australia) Early Career Fellowship funding (awarded to J.J., Application ID: APP1104745).

Acknowledgments: We would like to acknowledge and thank the Royal National Lifeboat Institution for their guidance and support.

Conflicts of Interest: The authors declare no conflict of interest. The funders had no role in the design of the study; in the collection, analyses, or interpretation of data; in the writing of the manuscript, or in the decision to publish the results.

Data Availability: Due to the qualitative nature of data collection, some participants may be identifiable from the contextual factors presented in the transcript. Data will be shared by the corresponding author on reasonable request.

References

1. Meddings, D.; Hyder, A.A.; Ozanne-Smith, J.; Rahman, A. *Global Report on Drowning: Preventing a Leading Killer*; World Health Organization: Geneva, Switzerland, 2014.
2. Menon, G.R.; Singh, L.; Sharma, P.; Yadav, P.; Singh, H.; Sati, P.; Begum, R.; Fadel, S.; Watson, L.; Jamison, D.T.; et al. National Burden Estimates of healthy life lost in India, 2017: An analysis using direct mortality data and indirect disability data. *Lancet Glob. Health* **2019**, *7*, e1675–e1684. [CrossRef]
3. Mahadevia Ghimire, K.; Vikas, M. Climate Change–Impact on the Sundarbans: A case study. *Int. Sci. J. Environ. Sci.* **2012**, *2*, 7–15.
4. Kanjilal, B.; Mazumdar, P.G.; Mukherjee, M.; Mondal, S.; Barman, D.; Singh, S.; Mandal, A. *Health Care in the Sundarbans (India): Challenges and Plan for a Better Future. Future Health Systems Research Programme*; Institute of Health Management Research: Jaipur, India, 2010.
5. Alonge, O.; Hyder, A.A. Reducing the global burden of childhood unintentional injuries. *Arch. Dis. Child.* **2014**, *99*, 62. [CrossRef] [PubMed]
6. Gupta, M.; Bhaumik, S.; Roy, S.; Panda, R.; Peden, M.; Jagnoor, J. Determining child drowning mortality in the Sundarbans, India: Applying the Community Knowledge Approach. *Inj. Prev.* **2020**. [CrossRef]

7. Lukaszyk, C.; Mittal, S.; Gupta, M.; Das, R.; Ivers, R.; Jagnoor, J. The impact and understanding of childhood drowning by a community in West Bengal, India, and the suggested preventive measures. *Acta Paediatr.* **2018**, *108*. [CrossRef]
8. Bogart, L.M.; Uyeda, K. Community-Based Participatory Research: Partnering with Communities for Effective and Sustainable Behavioral Health Interventions. *Health Psychol.* **2009**, *28*, 391–393. [CrossRef]
9. Hodge, L.M.; Turner, K.M.T. Sustained Implementation of Evidence-based Programs in Disadvantaged Communities: A Conceptual Framework of Supporting Factors. *Am. J. Community Psychol.* **2016**, *58*, 192–210. [CrossRef]
10. Wight, D.; Wimbush, E.; Jepson, R.; Doi, L. Six steps in quality intervention development (6SQuID). *J. Epidemiol. Community Health* **2016**, *70*, 520. [CrossRef]
11. Puri, S.; Fernandez, S.; Puranik, A.; Anand, D.; Syed, Z.; Patel, A.; Uddin, S.; Thow, A.M. Policy content and stakeholder network analysis for infant and young child feeding in India. *BMC Public Health* **2017**, *17*, 461. [CrossRef]
12. Gruen, R.L.; Elliott, J.H.; Nolan, M.L.; Lawton, P.D.; Parkhill, A.; McLaren, C.J.; Lavis, J.N. Sustainability science: An integrated approach for health-programme planning. *Lancet* **2008**, *372*, 1579–1589. [CrossRef]
13. Uzochukwu, B.; Onwujekwe, O.; Mbachu, C.; Okwuosa, C.; Etiaba, E.; Nyström, M.E.; Gilson, L. The challenge of bridging the gap between researchers and policy makers: Experiences of a Health Policy Research Group in engaging policy makers to support evidence informed policy making in Nigeria. *Glob. Health* **2016**, *12*, 67. [CrossRef] [PubMed]
14. Shiffman, J.; Smith, S. Generation of political priority for global health initiatives: A framework and case study of maternal mortality. *Lancet* **2007**, *370*, 9. [CrossRef]
15. Gupta, M.; Zwi, A.B.; Jagnoor, J. Opportunities for the development of drowning interventions in West Bengal, India: A review of policy and government programs. *BMC Public Health* **2020**, *20*, 704. [CrossRef] [PubMed]
16. Maity, B. Interstate differences in the performance of Anganwadi centres under ICDS scheme. *Econ. Polit. Wkly.* **2016**, *51*, 59–66.
17. Chatterjee, S.; Apartment, M. Self-help groups and economic empowerment of rural women: A case study. *Int. J. Educ. Manag. Stud.* **2014**, *4*, 103–107.
18. Scott, K.; Shanker, S. Tying their hands? Institutional obstacles to the success of the ASHA community Health Worker Programme Rural North India. *AIDS Care* **2010**, *22*, 1606–1612. [CrossRef]
19. Government of West Bengal. *State Plan of Action for Children (2014–18)*; Department of Child Development and Women Development & Social Welfare: West Bengal, India, 2014.
20. Tong, A.; Craig, J.; Sainsbury, P. Consolidated criteria for reporting qualitative research (COREQ): A 32-item checklist for interviews and focus groups. *Int. J. Qual. Health Care* **2007**, *19*, 349–357. [CrossRef]
21. NVivo Qualitative Data Analysis Software. Available online: https://www.qsrinternational.com/nvivo-qualitative-data-analysis-software/home (accessed on 25 June 2020).
22. Carter, N.; Bryant-Lukosius, D.; DiCenso, A.; Blythe, J.; Neville, A.J. The use of triangulation in qualitative research. *Oncol. Nurs. Forum* **2014**, *41*, 545–547. [CrossRef]
23. Mendelow, A.L. Environmental scanning: The impact of the stakeholder concept. In Proceedings of the Second International Conference on Information Systems, Cambridge, MA, USA, 7–9 December 1981.
24. World Health Organization. *Preventing Drowning: An Implementation Guide*; World Health Organization: Geneva, Switzerland, 2017.
25. Movsisyan, A.; Arnold, L.; Evans, R.; Hallingberg, B.; Moore, G.; O'Cathain, A.; Pfadenhauer, L.M.; Segrott, J.; Rehfuess, E. Adapting evidence-informed complex population health interventions for new contexts: A systematic review of guidance. *Implement Sci.* **2019**, *14*, 105. [CrossRef]
26. Mitchell, R.J.; Ryder, T. Rethinking the public health model for injury prevention. *Inj. Prev.* **2020**, *26*, 2. [CrossRef]
27. Cantwell, N.; Davidson, J.; Elsley, S.; Milligan, I.; Quinn, N. *Moving Forward: Implementing the 'Guidelines for the Alternative Care of Children'*; Centre for Excellence for Looked After Children in Scotland: Glasgow, UK, 2012.
28. United Nations General Assembly. *Guidelines for the Alternative Care of Children*; United Nations General Assembly: New York, NY, USA, 2010.
29. Lukaszyk, C.; Ivers, R.Q.; Jagnoor, J. Systematic review of drowning in India: Assessment of burden and risk. *Inj. Prev.* **2018**, *24*, 451–458. [CrossRef]

30. Harvey, B.; Stuart, J.; Swan, T. Evaluation of a Drama-in-Education Programme to Increase AIDS Awareness in South African High Schools: A Randomized Community Intervention Trial. *Int. J. STD AIDS* **2000**, *11*, 105–111. [CrossRef] [PubMed]
31. Gielen, A.C.; Sleet, D. Application of Behavior-Change Theories and Methods to Injury Prevention. *Epidemiol. Rev.* **2003**, *25*, 65–76. [CrossRef] [PubMed]
32. Tankard, M.E.; Paluck, E.L. Norm Perception as a Vehicle for Social Change. *Soc. Issues Policy Rev.* **2016**, *10*, 181–211. [CrossRef]
33. Ryan, R.M.; Patrick, H.; Deci, E.L.; Williams, G.C. Facilitating health behaviour change and its maintenance: Interventions based on self-determination theory. *Eur. Health Psychol.* **2008**, *10*, 2–5.
34. Kwasnicka, D.; Dombrowski, S.U.; White, M.; Sniehotta, F. Theoretical explanations for maintenance of behaviour change: A systematic review of behaviour theories. *Health Psychol. Rev.* **2016**, *10*, 277–296. [CrossRef] [PubMed]
35. Ved, R.; Scott, K.; Gupta, G.; Ummer, O.; Singh, S.; Srivastava, A.; George, A.S. How are gender inequalities facing India's one million ASHAs being addressed? Policy origins and adaptations for the world's largest all-female community health worker programme. *Hum. Resour. Health* **2019**, *17*, 3. [CrossRef]
36. Mondal, N.; Murhekar, M.V. Factors associated with low performance of Accredited Social Health Activist (ASHA) regarding maternal care in Howrah district, West Bengal, 2015–16: An unmatched case control study. *Clin. Epidemiol. Global Health* **2018**, *6*, 21–28. [CrossRef]
37. Frieden, T.R. Six Components Necessary for Effective Public Health Program Implementation. *Am. J. Public Health* **2013**, *104*, 17–22. [CrossRef] [PubMed]
38. Abimbola, S. Beyond positive a priori bias: Reframing community engagement in LMICs. *Health Promot. Int.* **2019**, *35*, 598–609. [CrossRef] [PubMed]
39. Bardhan, P.; Mookherjee, D. Pro-poor targeting and accountability of local governments in West Bengal. *J. Dev. Econ.* **2006**, *79*, 303–327. [CrossRef]
40. Odugleh-Koleva, A.; Parrish-Sprowl, J. Universal health coverage and community engagement. *Bull. World Health Organ.* **2018**, *96*, 589–664. [CrossRef] [PubMed]
41. Kok, M.C.; Broerse, J.E.W.; Theobald, S.; Ormel, H.; Dieleman, M.; Taegtmeyer, M. Performance of community health workers: Situating their intermediary position within complex adaptive health systems. *Human Resour. Health* **2017**, *15*, 59. [CrossRef] [PubMed]
42. El Arifeen, S.; Christou, A.; Reichenbach, L.; Osman, F.A.; Azad, K.; Islam, K.S.; Ahmed, F.; Perry, H.B.; Peters, D.H. Community-based approaches and partnerships: Innovations in health-service delivery in Bangladesh. *Lancet* **2013**, *382*, 2012. [CrossRef]
43. Bertone, M.P.; Lagarde, M.; Witter, S. Performance-based financing in the context of the complex remuneration of health workers: Findings from a mixed-method study in rural Sierra Leone. *BMC Health Serv. Res.* **2016**, *16*, 286. [CrossRef]
44. Bracht, N.; Finnegan, J.R., Jr.; Rissel, C.; Weisbrod, R.; Gleaso, J.; Corbett, J.; Veblen-Mortenson, S. Community ownership and program continuation following a health demonstration project. *Health Educ. Res.* **1994**, *9*, 243–255. [CrossRef]
45. Branche, C.; Ozanne-Smith, J.; Oyebite, K.; Hyder, A.A. *World Report on Child Injury Prevention*; World Health Organization: Geneva, Switzerland, 2008.
46. Violano, P.; Davis, K.A.; Lane, V.; Lofthouse, R.; Carusone, C. Establishing an Injury Prevention Program to Address Pediatric Pedestrian Collisions. *J. Trauma Nurs.* **2009**, *16*, 216–219. [CrossRef]
47. Cornwall, A.; Jewkes, R. What is participatory research? *Soc. Sci. Med.* **1995**, *41*, 1667–1676. [CrossRef]

48. Douthwaite, B.; Beaulieu, N.; Lundy, M.; Peters, D. Understanding how participatory approaches foster innovation. *Int. J. Agric. Sustain.* **2009**, *7*, 42–60. [CrossRef]
49. Thomas-Slayter, B. Participatory Approaches to Community Change: Building Cooperation through Dialogue and Negotiation Using Participatory Rural Appraisal. In *Handbook on Building Cultures of Peace*; De Rivera, J., Ed.; Springer: New York, NY, USA, 2009; pp. 333–348.

Publisher's Note: MDPI stays neutral with regard to jurisdictional claims in published maps and institutional affiliations.

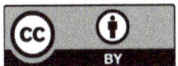

© 2020 by the authors. Licensee MDPI, Basel, Switzerland. This article is an open access article distributed under the terms and conditions of the Creative Commons Attribution (CC BY) license (http://creativecommons.org/licenses/by/4.0/).

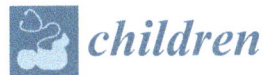

Article

Preventing Child Drowning in the Philippines: The Need to Address the Determinants of Health

Jonathan P. Guevarra [1,*], Amy E. Peden [2,3,4], Lita L. Orbillo [5], Maria Rosario Sylvia Z. Uy [5], Joseph John R. Madrilejos [5], John Juliard L. Go [6], Rammell Eric C. Martinez [6], Lolita L. Cavinta [7] and Richard C Franklin [2,3]

[1] Department of Health Promotion and Education, College of Public Health, University of the Philippines Manila, 625 Pedro Gil St., Ermita, Manila 1000, Philippines
[2] College of Public Health, Medical and Veterinary Sciences, James Cook University, Townsville, QLD 4811, Australia; a.peden@unsw.edu.au (A.E.P.); richard.franklin@jcu.edu.au (R.C.F.)
[3] Royal Life Saving Society—Australia, Broadway, NSW 2581, Australia
[4] School of Population Health, University of New South Wales, Kensington, NSW 2033, Australia
[5] Disease Prevention and Control Bureau, Department of Health, Sta. Cruz, Manila 1003, Philippines; litaorbillo_rn@yahoo.com (L.L.O.); herb_ross@yahoo.com (M.R.S.Z.U.); josephjohnmadrilejos@gmail.com (J.J.R.M.)
[6] World Health Organization, Office of the Representative in the Philippines, Sta. Cruz, Manila 1003, Philippines; GoJ@who.int (J.J.L.G.); rmartinez@who.int (R.E.C.M.)
[7] University of the Philippines-College of Public Health Foundation, Inc., 625 Pedro Gil St., Ermita, Manila 1000, Philippines; lolitacavinta@gmail.com
* Correspondence: jpguevarra2@up.edu.ph; Tel.: +63-25-260-811

Received: 9 December 2020; Accepted: 28 December 2020; Published: 7 January 2021

Abstract: Drowning is a public health issue in the Philippines, with children at significantly increased risk. Determinants of health (DoH) such as education, socio-economic status, ethnicity, and urbanization are factors that impact drowning risk. As drowning is a multisectoral issue, a national drowning prevention plan can drive collaboration with relevant stakeholders. This study reports trends in unintentional child (0–14 years) drowning in the Philippines (incidence, rates, and trends over time for fatal and non-fatal (years lived with a disability (YLDs) and disability adjusted life years (DALYs) from 2008–2017 and conducts an analysis of the Philippines' Multisector Action Plan (MSAP) on Drowning Prevention. From 2008–2017, 27,928 (95%UI [Uncertainty Interval]: 22,794–33,828) children aged 0–14 years died from drowning (52.7% aged 5–14 years old). Rates of drowning have declined among both age groups, with greater reductions seen among 0–4 year olds (y = −0.3368x + 13.035; $R^2 = 0.9588$). The MSAP has 12 child drowning-specific activities and 20 activities were identified where DoH will need to be considered during development and implementation. The MSAP activities, and work done to prevent drowning more generally, must consider DoH such as education, urbanization, water and sanitation health, and safe water transportation. A national drowning surveillance system and investment in research in the Philippines are recommended.

Keywords: child; drowning; water; safety; prevention; mortality; policy; stakeholder; Global Burden of Disease; multisector

1. Introduction

Drowning in low- and middle-income countries has been identified as an issue requiring significant investment in order to reduce the burden to global public health [1]. Around the world, 295,000 people are estimated to die from unintentional drowning annually [2], with the true burden likely to be significantly higher when including transportation and disaster-related drowning [3]. The vast majority of drowning occurs in low- and middle-income countries and children are most at risk [1]. Fatal drowning ranks as the 13th leading cause of death among children under 15 years of age, with the 1–4 years age group at greatest risk [4]. Child drowning rates in low- and middle-income countries are six times higher than those in high-income countries [5].

Reducing child drowning is an area of key focus for the drowning prevention community. Across decades of research the risk factors for child drowning are reasonably well understood [5–7]. These include a lack of supervision when children are in or around water, unrestricted access to water through the absence of barriers or covers such as for wells, lack of awareness of dangers owing to their young age, and an inability to swim [8–10]. Quick rescue and resuscitation in instances of drowning are context dependent, with quick rescue and appropriate medical care a significant factor in survival [11]. What is less well understood is what influences the uptake of these strategies given that drowning often impacts those from low socio-economic backgrounds [1].

The Philippines is a developing country in the Western Pacific region that has made progress in reducing child mortality over past decades. Between 1990 and 2015, deaths of infants under one year decreased from 41 to 21 per 1000 live births, while the number of children who died before the age of five dropped from 59 to 27 per 1000 live births. However, determinants of health impact progress. Childhood immunization rates are low and in some cases declining, leading to increased incidence of vaccine-preventable diseases [12]. Children and adolescents in the Philippines have limited access to sexual and reproductive health services, with recent teen fertility rates now at levels comparable to the 1960s [12]. Children and youth aged 13–24 years in the Philippines experience high levels of physical (64%), psychological (62%), sexual (22%), and peer (65%) violence [12].

Despite some encouraging progress in recent years, there are still limitations to children's access to education in the Philippines [12], a key determinant of health. As of 2015, 83.4% (primary) and around 73.9% (secondary) of enrolled children actually completed their schooling. In its 3rd National Plan of Action for Children (2017–2022), the Council for the Welfare of Children outlined a plan for improving child health and well-being, including access to education [13]. Similarly, the Philippines Department of Health outlines a range of national objectives for improving the health for children that includes reducing infant mortality and reducing injury-related deaths, specifically road traffic deaths [14].

Drowning, another cause of injury-related death, is a significant issue in the Philippines [15]. As a nation, the Philippines is an archipelago made up of 7107 islands and has an estimated 2019 population of 108,116,615 [16]. Due to the country's geography, exposure to water, and thus risk of drowning, is a daily occurrence [17]. It is estimated that an average of 3276 deaths due to accidental drowning occurred in the Philippines between 2006 and 2013, a rate of 3.5 per 100,000 population [18]. Children aged 0–14 years are a leading age group for drowning, with children 1–4 years at most risk [18]. Population density, large average household size, increasing urbanization, and a lack of piped water are determinants of health that contribute to increased drowning risk in the Philippines [19,20].

Drowning in the Philippines, as it is in other nations, is a public health issue that crosses multiple policy areas and agendas [21]. This is both positive and negative as there are multiple opportunities for political engagement and ways of framing the issue of drowning prevention. However, this may also mean that there is no clear leadership on the issue and no government ownership of the problem. As a means of gaining national traction on the issue of drowning prevention, the World Health Organization (WHO) proposes the capture, collation, and analysis of quality data on drowning and the development of water safety plans (in this article referred to as a drowning prevention plan) as two key pillars [22]. In response to this call to action, this study presents the most recent estimates for child drowning-related mortality and morbidity in the Philippines, as well as an analysis of the recently developed multisector action plan on drowning prevention in the Philippines, with a specific focus on children and determinants of health.

2. Materials and Methods

This study took a two-phase approach. Firstly, a retrospective study exploring unintentional drowning data for the Philippines for children 0–14 years of was accessed from the Global Burden of Disease (GBD) GBD Compare Viz Hub [23]. Within the context of the child drowning issue as depicted by the data, this study then aimed to document the process of, and results associated with, the development of a multisector action plan on drowning prevention in the Philippines.

2.1. Fatal and Non-Fatal Drowning Data in the Philippines

Data on unintentional drowning as a cause of death (C.2.2. Drowning derived from International Classification of Diseases [ICD] 9 and ICD10 code W65-74) were sourced from the GBD Compare Viz Hub for the Philippines. Data were accessed for children aged 0–14 years (age groups < 5 years and 5–14 years) between 2008 and 2017 (the latest publicly available data). Incidence and rates per 100,000 population were reported with a 95% uncertainty interval (UI). Trends over time were explored using a linear trend as calculated in Microsoft Excel. Data were explored by sex, age group, and by year of drowning fatality. Non-fatal drowning data were reported using Years Lost due to Disability (YLDs). The overall burden of child drowning in the Philippines is expressed through disability adjusted life years (DALYs). DALYs can be considered as 'one lost year of healthy life' and are calculated as the sum of the Years of Life Lost (YLL) due to premature mortality in the population and the YLD for people living with the health condition or its consequences [24].

2.2. Multisector Action Plan on Drowning Prevention

Recognizing that drowning is also one of the health issues that the Philippines needs to address, the country started working on the multisector action plan on drowning prevention in 2016.

2.2.1. Development of the Plan

The process of developing the action plan was guided by the global public health documents and commitments and by the Philippine health policies. [1,25–28]. The Department of Health, in collaboration with various institutions led by the World Health Organization and with support from the Bloomberg Philanthropies, developed the Multisector Action Plan on Drowning Prevention in the Philippines, 2016–2026.

Core group meetings, attended by representatives from the Department of Health of the Philippines, World Health Organization, and College of Public Health—University of the Philippines Manila, were held in preparation for conducting consultative meetings (Figure 1).

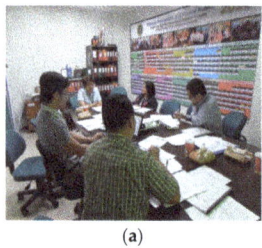 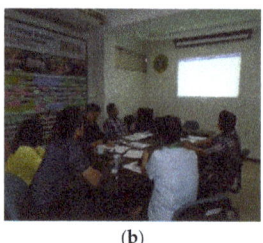 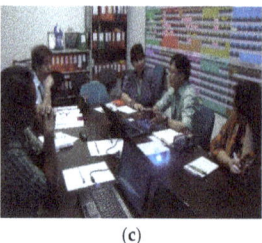

(a) (b) (c)

Figure 1. Core group meetings among the representatives of the University of the Philippines College of Public Health Foundation, Inc. [UP-CPHFI], Department of Health (DOH), and World Health Organization (WHO): (**a**) Initial planning on how to conduct the multisector action plan development; (**b**) discussion of the agenda and activities for the multi action plan development; (**c**) discussion on the proceedings of the multisector action plan development.

Five consultative meetings with various stakeholders were held. The participants in the consultative meetings were from Department of Health (DOH), World Health Organization (WHO), National Economic and Development Authority (NEDA), Department of Education (DepEd), Philippine Coast Guard (PCG), Maritime Industry Authority (MARINA), Philippine Red Cross (PRC), Safe Kids Worldwide Philippines, National Youth Commission (NYC), National Council for Disability Affairs (NCDA), Office of Civil Defense (OCD), Department of Interior and Local Government (DILG), Department of Tourism (DOT), Philippine College of Emergency Medicine (PCEM), University of the Philippines College of Public Health Foundation, Inc. (UP-CPHFI), Council for the Welfare of Children (CWC), Philippine National Police (PNP), Philippine Statistics Authority (PSA), Philippine Information Agency (PIA), and the Philippine Lifesaving Society (PLS) (Figure 2).

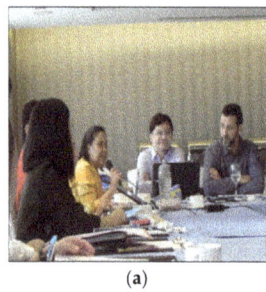 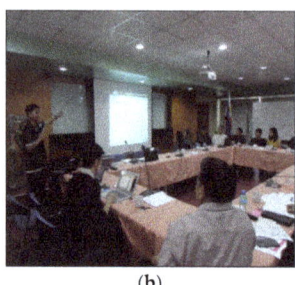 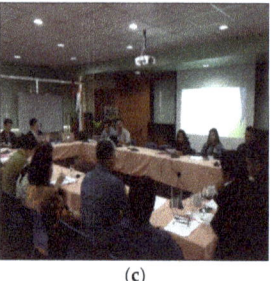

(a) (b) (c)

Figure 2. Consultative meetings: (**a**) Multisector action plan meeting with Dr. David Meddings of the WHO; (**b**) presentation of drowning prevention activities being implemented by one agency; (**c**) discussion on the contents of the Multisector Action Plan on Drowning Prevention.

The multisector action plan on drowning prevention was presented during the Violence and Injury Prevention Program (VIPP) Forum. This forum was attended by representatives from various organizations (government, non-government, and civil society organizations). This forum also served as a public hearing on the multisector action plan (Figure 3). Finally, the plan was presented in a "Partners' Meeting on Drowning Prevention in the Philippines" in February 2017.

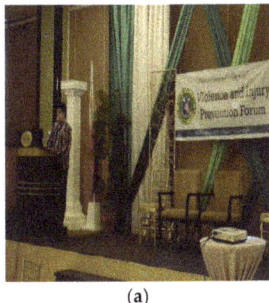 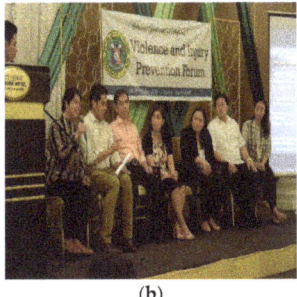 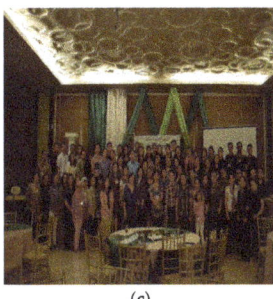

Figure 3. Public hearing on the Multisector Action Plan on Drowning Prevention in the Philippines: (**a**) presentation of the Multisector Plan on Drowning Prevention in the Philippines, 2016–2026; (**b**) panel addressing questions from the participants; (**c**) group photo of the participants who attended the public hearing.

2.2.2. Analysis of the Plan

The activities of the multisector action plan on drowning prevention in the Philippines were analyzed to identify those activities relevant to child or youth drowning prevention and to identify activities where social determinants of health need to be considered when delivering the activity. Analyses were performed by consensus among the authors. Each author coded the activities separately and disagreements were discussed until consensus was achieved.

2.3. Ethics Approvals

This study used publicly accessible, de-identified data and as such did not require institutional ethics board approval. Similarly, the process of developing the multisector action plan on drowning was also deemed exempt from requiring ethics approval.

3. Results

This section outlines data trends in child drowning in the Philippines while also exploring the multisector action plan relevant to child drowning reduction and the determinants of health.

3.1. Child Drowning Deaths in the Philippines

In total, 27,928 (95% Uncertainty Interval [UI]: 22,794–33,828) children aged 0–14 years died from drowning in the Philippines between 2008 and 2017 (Table 1). Fatal drowning among 5–14 year old children accounted for 52.7% of all deaths among the 0–14 years age group.

Table 1. Number of drowning deaths by year and age group, children 0–14 years, Philippines, 2008–2017.

	0–4 Years (95% UI)	5–14 Years (95% UI)	Total 0–14 Years (95% UI)
2008	1436 (1145–1800)	1507 (1330–1714)	2943 (2474–3514)
2009	1416 (1149–1738)	1529 (1340–1735)	2944 (2489–3472)
2010	1384 (1122–1684)	1510 (1322–1727)	2899 (2444–3411)
2011	1393 (1097–1710)	1513 (1317–1738)	2905 (2414–3448)
2012	1364 (1028–1732)	1506 (1303–1741)	2869 (2332–3473)
2013	1330 (975–1731)	1459 (1259–1684)	2789 (2234–3415)
2014	1318 (956–1729)	1450 (1236–1689)	2768 (2192–3417)
2015	1283 (933–1669)	1483 (1255–1749)	2766 (2188–3418)
2016	1180 (888–1506)	1424 (1193–1696)	2605 (2082–3202)
2017	1110 (842–1436)	1329 (1104–1622)	2439 (1946–3058)
Total	13,214 (10.135–16,735)	14,714 (12,659–17,093)	27,928 (22,794–33,828)

Rates of child drowning for both age groups declined over the study period, with drowning among 0–4 year olds declining at a faster pace (y = −0.3368x + 13.035; R^2 = 0.9588) than 0–14 year olds (y = −0.0634x + 7.3047; R^2 = 0.5252) (Figure 4). Among 0–4 year olds, rates varied from a high of 12.67 per 100,000 children to a current low of 9.30 per 100,000 population in 2017; whereas rates for 5–14 year olds varied from a high of 7.15 per 100,000 population to a low of 6.29.

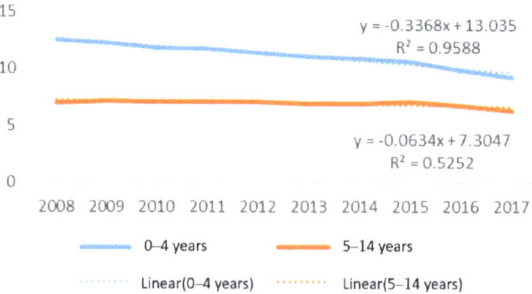

Figure 4. Trends over time in rate of fatal drowning per 100,000 population, 0–4 years and 5–14 years age groups, Philippines, 2008–2017.

When examined by sex, males aged both 0–4 years old and 5–14 years old recorded higher rates of drowning when compared to females. Male drowning rates among 0–4 year olds varied from a high of 15.09 per 100,000 population in 2008 to a low of 11.20 in 2017, compared to a rate of 9.88 in 2008 and 7.26 in 2017 for females. For 5–14 year olds, drowning rates for males varied from a high of 8.94 in 2015 to a current low of 7.86 in 2017, whereas female drowning rates varied from a high of 5.32 in 2011 to a current low of 4.62 per 100,000 in 2017. Male drowning rates among the 0–4 years and 5–14 years age groups declined at a faster pace than females (0–4 years: males $y = -0.4018x + 15.726$; $R^2 = 0.9453$; females $y = -0.2679x + 10.157$; $R^2 = 0.9752$; 5–14 years: males $y = -0.0626x + 9.0073$; $R^2 = 0.3567$; females $y = -0.0659x + 5.5033$; $R^2 = 0.7285$). (Figure 5).

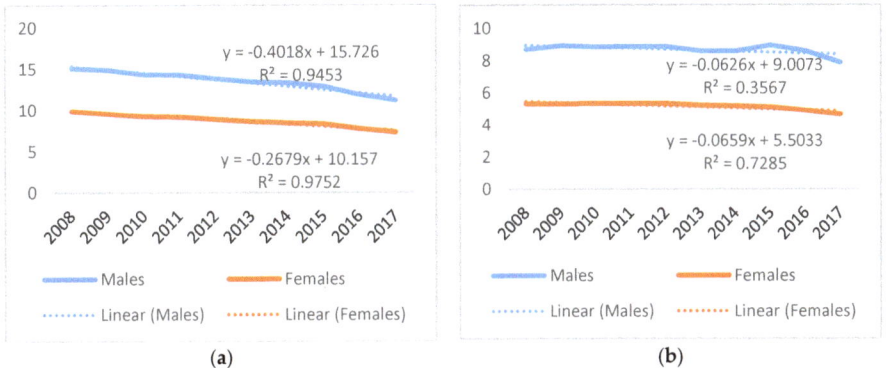

Figure 5. Fatal unintentional drowning rates per 100,000 population and sex, Philippines, 2008–2017: (**a**) 0–4 year olds, males' and females' rate and linear trend; (**b**) 5–14 year olds, males' and females' rate and linear trend.

When examining data on non-fatal child drowning in the Philippines, a total of 2267.7 YLDs were recorded for children 0–14 years in the Philippines across the study period. Children aged 5–14 years accounted for 83.7% ($n = 1898.9$) of the child drowning total burden (Figure 6).

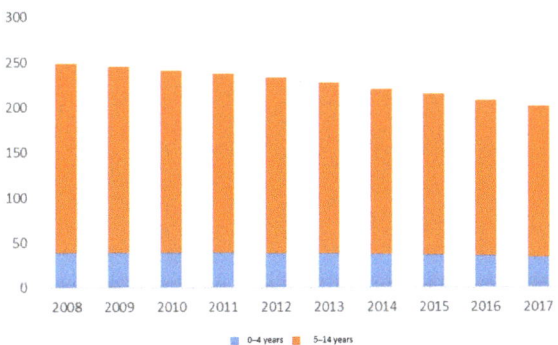

Figure 6. Years of Life Lost to Disability due to drowning by age group, Philippines 2008–2017.

For the total burden of drowning among children aged 0–14 years in the Philippines, there were a total of 2,292,471.0 DALYs recorded across the study period. The DALYs burden is evenly split between the age groups, with 5–14 year olds accounting for 50.6% of the total burden. When examining trends over time, the unintentional drowning-related DALY burden declined for both age groups, with a more significant decline over the study period in the 0–4 years age group (y = −2776.3x + 128512; R^2 = 0.8754) (Figure 7).

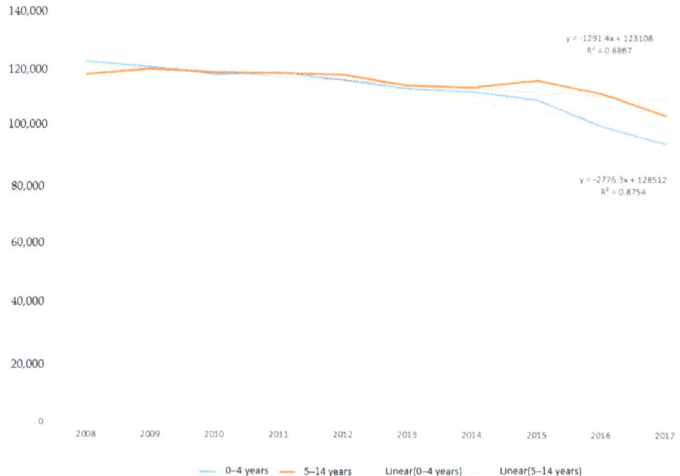

Figure 7. Number of Disability Adjusted Life Years (DALYs) for unintentional drowning and linear trend by age group, children 0–14 years, Philippines, 2008–2017.

3.2. Multisector Action Plan on Drowning Prevention

The multisector action plan on drowning prevention has two guiding principles, namely: Health IN ALL (i.e., Health in All Policies) and Health BY ALL (i.e., Whole of Government and Whole of Society). These principles underpin an overall goal of reducing the drowning mortality rate in the Philippines by 50% by the year 2026. The multisector action plan on drowning prevention outlines five objectives, underpinned by 16 strategies and 53 activities, to achieve its goal. There are a range of objectives that include activities specifically targeting child drowning prevention. There were 12 activities identified by the authors as being child-specific and 20 activities where determinants of health will need to be considered when undertaking the activities. (Table 2)

Table 2. Activities of the Multisector Action Plan on Drowning Prevention in the Philippines 2016–2026, relevance to children and consideration of determinants of health (DoH).

Activities	Child-Specific	DoH
Objective 1. To strengthen multisectoral collaboration on drowning prevention		
Strategy 1: Alliance building (Formation of Violence and Injury Prevention Alliance—VIPA)		
Multisectoral stakeholder meetings		
Operationalization of the multisectoral action plan on drowning prevention		✓
Formulation of the Joint Memorandum Circular between and among government agencies		
Integration of Drowning Prevention in the National Plan of Action for Children	✓	
Integration of drowning prevention in the Philippine Youth Development Plan	✓	✓
Integration of drowning prevention in the Philippine Development Plan for 2022		
Conduct drowning prevention strategic planning cum write shop with the end goal of crafting a dedicated Drowning Prevention Plan per participating Local Government Units (LGU)		
Strategy 2: Advocacy (Inclusion of drowning prevention plan in regional, local government and sectoral development plans; legislation)		
Advocating for and mobilization of resources from donor partners		
Creation of policy briefs for advocacy on drowning prevention among school-age children	✓	✓
Inclusion of drowning prevention in celebration of the National Disability Prevention and Rehabilitation (NDPR) Week and other special events		✓
Objective 2: To enhance interventions on drowning prevention especially in high-risk groups		
Strategy 1: Constant adult supervision		
Inclusion of and giving emphasis on constant adult supervision in communication materials	✓	✓
Strategy 2: Barriers		
Installation of barriers in areas that are prone to drowning	✓	✓
Strategy 3: Capability-building		
Training on Violence and Injury Prevention and Basic Life Support (BLS) to Violence and Injury Prevention focal persons and centers for health development managers		✓
Conduct of First Aid and BLS Cardiopulmonary Resuscitation (CPR), Accident Prevention, Ambulance Services, Learn to Swim, Lifeguarding, Swift Water Rescue, Water Search and Rescue (WASAR)		✓
Conduct of Training for Seafarers		
Conduct of Community-Based Disability-Inclusive Disaster Risk Reduction and Management		✓
Integration of Standardized Drowning management in the Technical Education and Skills Development Authority (TESDA) National Training Regulations of EMT-B.		
Training of tourist police on First Aid		
Learn to Swim and Survive	✓	✓
Strategy 4: Pre-hospital care emergency medical system		
Lobbying for the Passage of the Emergency Medical Service Systems (EMS) bill		
Development of guidelines for prehospital EMS		
Establishment of the pre-hospital EMS and expansion to other areas and LGUs		✓
Development and integration of standards for management of Drowning, submersion incidents, and Decompression illness in pre-hospital and Emergency department protocols.		

Table 2. Cont.

Activities	Child-Specific	DoH
Objective 3: To strengthen implementation and enforcement of policies and regulations on Drowning prevention		
Strategy 1: Strengthening of regulations on safety of beachgoers and related equipment and facilities		
Enforcement of guidelines for safety and security requirements for coastal and beach resorts, and vessels with pool facilities including qualification of lifeguards		
Enforcement of the guidelines for the operation of recreational watercrafts		✓
Enforcement of the guidelines on conducting marine parades, regattas, and other maritime-related activities		
Strategy 2: Use of flotation devices		
Enforcement of vessel safety inspection		
Pre-departure inspection of vessel		
Development of standards for flotation devices		
Strategy 3: Transport policies and regulations		
Establishment of traffic separation system in dense areas		✓
Establishment of Vessel Traffic Management System (VTMS)		
Conduct of compliance monitoring of ships and motorized bancas nationwide		
Investigation and appropriate recommendations on all maritime accidents in the Philippines		
Strategy 4: Policies and regulations related to weather disturbances		
Enforcement of No-Sail policy during inclement weather		
Contingency planning on typhoon and storm surge		
Objective 4: To increase public awareness on drowning prevention		
Strategy 1: Information dissemination activities (using various platforms)		
Development of health promotion, advocacy and communication materials on drowning prevention		✓
Utilization of Social Media in disseminating messages on drowning prevention		✓
Provide communication and information dissemination assistance and Dissemination of Information, Education and communication (IEC) materials		✓
Creation of support instructional materials for teachers or reference materials to be utilized in the classroom	✓	
Development of advocacy materials on child safety including drowning	✓	
Provision of publicity assistance in the implementation of the Drowning Prevention Program		
Promotion in the Regional Youth Advisory Council	✓	✓
Distribution of the "Drowning Safety Tips" to all beneficiary schools	✓	
Strategy 2: Conferences, seminars and community sessions on drowning prevention		
Conduct of conferences on drowning prevention		✓
Conduct of seminars on drowning prevention in educational institutions	✓	
Strategy 3: Advocacy (Drowning Prevention Consciousness Week)		
Issuance of Proclamation on the annual celebration of Drowning Consciousness Week		
Issuance of memo by Department of Education field offices on celebration of Drowning Consciousness Week	✓	

Table 2. *Cont.*

Activities	Child-Specific	DoH
Objective 5: To improve evidence and data on drowning		
Strategy 1: Information-sharing		
Collection of data on drowning on regular basis		
Preparation of disaggregated data of drowning		✓
Strategy 2: Strengthening of information management systems		
Establishment of continuous surveillance		
Enhancement of Injury Surveillance System (ISS) through personnel augmentation and review of the definitions or the data dictionary of the injury type		
Strategy 3: Implementation of research on drowning and drowning prevention		
Inclusion of drowning-related studies in the National Health Research Agenda		
Conduct of research activities on drowning and drowning prevention.		✓

Notes: DoH = Social Determinants of Health.

4. Discussion

Drowning is a leading, yet preventable, cause of child death [2,5,7,19]. While risk factors for child drowning are well understood [8–10], greater consideration of the impact of determinants of health on drowning risk are needed, as well as greater investment in upstream strategies that will contribute to reducing this risk. This study explored child drowning in the Philippines, through epidemiological analysis of country-level data and an assessment of the multisector action plan on drowning prevention's relevance to children within the context of determinants of health. These two areas of focus of this study reflect two of the key elements of the WHO Implementation Guide for drowning prevention—namely, quality data on drowning and a national water safety plan [22].

4.1. The Importance of Data on Drowning

Drowning is a key concern in the Philippines, with an age-standardized, cause-specific mortality rate of 5.30 per 100,000 people, 17% higher than the average for middle-income countries globally (4.30 per 100,000) [2]. Although the drowning rate in the Philippines has been decreasing, there is a need for increased action to speed the reduction in drowning deaths and there are a number of strategies that have been shown to be effective [29–33]. The reduction in drowning deaths was more pronounced with the 0–4 year olds, indicating further work is required in finding age-appropriate strategies to prevent drowning among 5–14 year olds.

While reductions in drowning among children are pleasing, it must be noted that the Global Burden of Disease estimates for drowning exclude incidents as a result of disasters and transportation [3]. This is likely to significantly underreport drowning in the Philippines given the impact of disasters such as typhoons and flooding [34], as well as the significant amount of inter-island travel that is conducted on boats and ferries [35].

4.2. Multisectoral Collaboration on Drowning Prevention (Objective 1)

Addressing the determinants of health that impact drowning require a multisectoral approach [1,21]. The development of the multisector action plan on drowning prevention in the Philippines was guided by principles from policy documents both international (Health in All Policies (HiAP), Whole-of-Government, and Whole-of-Society approaches) and local policy guidelines. HiAP is an approach to public policies across sectors that systematically takes into account the health implications of decisions, seeks synergies, and avoids harmful health impacts in order to improve population health and health equity. It improves accountability of policymakers for health impacts at all levels of policy-making. It includes an emphasis on the consequences of public policies on health systems, determinants of health, and well-being. The Whole-of-Government Approach invokes a participative endeavor among the different national government agencies for health, education, sports, environment, urban planning, transportation and communication, labor and employment, industry and trade, finance, energy, agriculture, and social development, among many possible others.

Another strength noted is the participation of various public agencies and non-government organizations in developing the Multisector Action Plan on Drowning Prevention in the Philippines. The participants of the collaborative effort to develop the action plan on drowning prevention have incorporated some recommendations made by the WHO-Regional Office for the Western Pacific (WPRO) when it comes to organizations that must be involved in such an undertaking [26]. However, there is always a need to exert effort and to collaborate more with other agencies that can provide data, share their interventions on drowning prevention (such as disaster response and transport), and provide the needed support in order to implement interventions aimed at reducing child drowning deaths (such as planning and development, and finance sectors). This sensible and needed approach recognizes and allows all agencies to be involved in drowning prevention, although this is not without challenges due to shifting priorities and staff movement. However, it is worth mentioning that the "coming together" of various organizations, with their own agency mandates and activities, has willingly contributed in meaningful discussions on how to address the drowning problem in the Philippines.

As of 2020, several agencies have already agreed to carry their specific agency commitments, with only a few remaining agencies having not yet agreed to implement commitments due to reasons such as changes in agency leadership resulting in a change in agency representative. One good thing is that, even though there have been changes in the composition of the multisector group, attendance and discussions on how to move forward has been maintained.

The Whole-of-Society Approach invokes the participation of government agencies, non-government agencies, private sector, business sector, and academia. The Philippine Health Agenda (PHA), seeking to fulfill the global call for Universal Health Coverage, adopting "All for Health towards Health for All" as the rallying point to realize the vision of a Healthy Philippines by 2022 [36], identifies that drowning prevention is required to achieve this goal. As identified in the multisector action plan on drowning prevention plan, there is also an opportunity to ensure that drowning prevention as an issue is embedded within plans and strategies of other sectors, such as ensuring drowning is identified in future iterations of the National Plan of Action for Children, the Philippines Youth Development Plan, and the Philippines Development Plan.

Education is a key determinant of health and, therefore, collaboration with Departments of Education will be required. Studies have shown school attendance to be protective for drowning, with higher rates of drowning seen during periods where children do not attend school (i.e., school holidays) [37]. Similarly, in Bangladesh, poorer education levels are linked to increased risk of drowning [31]. Education is also linked to socio-economic status, another determinant of health. Studies show children of low socio-economic backgrounds are at higher risk of drowning [37–41]. Ensuring all children have access to education will contribute to better health and well-being [42], as well as reduced drowning risk.

Other countries have instigated compulsory swimming lessons for school-aged children [41,43–45] to help address increasing the number of people with swimming skills and knowledge. This strategy is not without its own challenges as access to places to undertake learning to swim, school attendance, number of swim teachers, logistics of moving children from school and back again, and cost all place barriers to the delivery of school-based learn-to-swim programs [46,47].

Proximity to water is a key risk factor [7,19] and designing public works to help remove water hazards, such as open drains, building walkways over water for children going to school, and putting barriers in place so children cannot access water will all contribute to reducing drowning risk, thus engaging with the water, sanitation, and hygiene (WASH) community will also be required.

4.3. Interventions on Drowning Prevention Especially in High-Risk Groups (Objective 2)

The Philippines is a multicultural nation with many ethnic minorities. Such groups are shown to be at higher risk of drowning and have unique needs when it comes to reducing this risk [48,49]. Understanding the unique needs of these groups will be vital to ensuring the effective implementation of drowning prevention strategies. Identifying high-risk groups ensures the greatest impact of the plan and this objective proposes four strategies while also building on objective 1. Of these four strategies within objective 2, three directly target children (adult supervision, barriers, and learn to swim). However, for these activities to be successful the impact of the determinants of health will need to be considered.

Constant adult supervision is not a simple task, with the adult required to be within arm's reach, focused with all their attention, all of the time [8,50]; it also requires the adult to be prepared to supervise, which includes having necessary items with them so they do not need to leave the location (e.g., towels), an understanding of the child's skill level in the water, and reduction in distractions from other sources. Education, family size, culture, and financial circumstance all influence supervision and need to be part of the communication strategy.

Physical barriers separate a child from a water hazard to reduce drowning risk [51]. In the Philippines, barriers such as house/door barriers, porch barriers, barriers preventing children from going to creeks, and reconstructing or placing covers on open, dug wells as a form of barrier have been used in order to prevent younger children from exposure to hazards from their sources of water [19,52]. WASH reduces drowning risk. Having a piped water system can also solve concerns associated with getting water from open, dug wells, thereby eliminating exposure to drowning-prone areas. Installing barriers controlling access to water has also been recommended by the World Health Organization to reduce drowning risk [22].

In terms of capability-building strategy, it is envisioned that the younger population will be able to learn the basic swimming skills. However, this will require careful planning since children will be exposed to bodies of water, which is also a drowning risk. The recommended age for children to be exposed to swimming must also be carefully studied. Agencies involved in training different walks of life in swimming include the Philippine Coast Guard (PCG) and non-government organizations such as the Philippine Red Cross (PRC), Philippine Lifesaving Society (PLS), and Bert Lozada Foundation, Inc. to name a few. However, learn-to-swim programs for children have been implemented in other countries and have been noted to be worthwhile endeavors that low- and middle-income countries (LMICs) like the Philippines can learn from [43,53]. On another note, teaching school-age children (aged over 6 years) swimming and water safety skills is one of the recommended interventions to reduce drowning [22].

Other strategies such as learning CPR, which is not specifically targeted at children, has been recognized as a tertiary prevention strategy for saving children/people who have drowned [54]. Globally increasing CPR skills is a challenge and requires a wide range of strategies to ensure capture of the widest possible proportion of the population and will require an understanding of the determinants to ensure these strategies are effective [53]. Linking the requirement for CPR to another life event, such as leaving school, gaining a driver's license, etc., have been proposed as strategies to increase CPR uptake [55,56] and these should be considered in the Philippines.

4.4. Strengthening Implementation and Enforcement of Policies and Regulations on Drowning Prevention (Objective 3)

There were no activities that were directed at children in this objective. However, we note that floatation devices have been used elsewhere [57,58] to protect children when recreating in water. Lifesaving and rescue services can also help increase the safety of children by ensuring that the location where they recreate in the water is safe and they are able to be rescued if they get into trouble. Unfortunately, anecdotally, lifesaving services are more likely to be at resorts and tourist areas used by non-locals.

Rescue services for boating-related incidents have been found elsewhere [59] to help reduce drowning and these services are often used during times of disaster [60]. Agencies, such as the Philippine Coast Guard (PCG), Maritime Industry Authority (MARINA), and the Philippine National Police (PNP), have a very big role in providing rescue services, thereby contributing to the reduction of drowning incidents. Policies and regulations to improve occupational fishers have wider effects than just reducing drowning. Families of fishers will be protected if the fisher is protected, i.e., if the breadwinner of the family drowns, there are major economic and societal impacts on the family and broader community as a study from Tanzania showed [61].

4.5. Public Awareness on Drowning Prevention (Objective 4)

Strategies, and their associated activities, within this objective targeting child drowning prevention are information dissemination activities using various platforms (creation of instructional support materials for teachers or reference materials to be utilized in the classroom; development of advocacy materials on child safety including drowning, promotion of drowning prevention in the Regional Youth Advisory Council, and distribution of the 'Drowning Safety Tips' to all beneficiary schools). This should be undertaken using a health promotion approach that engages with the community and ensures messages are delivered in a manner and at a time that has the most impact.

Several agencies committed to contribute specific actions in order to increase public awareness on drowning prevention. To name a few, the Department of Health (DOH) together with the Department of Health Promotion of Education of the College of Public Health, University of the Philippines Manila (DHPE, CPH, UPM) will develop the health promotion, advocacy, and communication plans on drowning; the Philippine Information Agency (PIA) will assist in the dissemination of information, education, and communication (IEC) materials; the Department of Education (DepEd) will intensify the integration of drowning prevention in the K to 12 curriculum; the Council for the Welfare of Children will develop advocacy materials on child safety including drowning prevention; the National Youth Commission (NYC) will promote drowning prevention in the Regional Youth Advisory Council and in their social media campaigns. Other partner agencies will also contribute by promoting drowning prevention messages through social media (Philippine Red Cross), doing advocacy on drowning prevention in celebration of the National Disability Prevention and Rehabilitation (National Council for Disability Affairs); distributing IEC materials and conducting seminars to residents of coastal areas about safety tips regarding drowning prevention (Philippine National Police); distributing the "Drowning Safety Tips" to all beneficiary schools and conducting social media campaigns on drowning prevention (Safe Kids Worldwide Philippines). The school is one of the best places to advocate drowning prevention. With the support of the educational sector, the officials, administrators, and the student body, it is hoped that a policy for the institutionalization on the celebration of Drowning Consciousness Week can be crafted and implemented.

Increasing public awareness through the conduct of seminars in educational institutions is also a very important activity that is directed to the younger population groups. The WHO has also recommended to strengthen public awareness of drowning through strategic communications to support drowning prevention interventions. Drowning prevention messages and materials can be disseminated through various platforms [22].

4.6. Evidence and Data on Drowning (Objective 5)

A challenge facing those working to prevent child drowning globally, including in the Philippines, is a lack of timely, quality data [4,22]. GBD data, as were used in this study, are modeled data and may be inaccessible to researchers and drowning prevention advocates. GBD data also lack information about risk factors such as activity and location as well as the presence or absence of prevention strategies (for example, the wearing of life jackets) to help inform stratagems to redress the drowning burden. Further work needs to be undertaken to ensure quality data capture on fatal and non-fatal drowning at the country level, with data made available to those who need it, which is comprehensive and helps inform drowning prevention. The first steps toward better data have been undertaken with the development of Online National Electronic Injury Surveillance System (ONEISS), a national injury (including drowning) surveillance system in the Philippines. ONEISS data can be used as the source of information in determining primary cause and risk factors of drowning [62]. However, there are limitations for using the ONEISS data as (1) the data are collected by selected hospitals, (2) the system is web based and hospitals with no or poor access to the internet will have problems in using the system, (3) drowning events captured by local health clinics are not usually reported, (4) cataclysmic events and water transport accidents are not included, and (5), like other countries in Asia, misclassification of cases could be a problem. The role of the Philippine Statistics Authority (PSA) in collecting timely and complete data cannot be overemphasized. In addition, there may be a need for government agencies such as the Philippine Coast Guard (PCG), Department of Health (DOH), and Philippine Statistics Authority (PSA) to sit down and further discuss how data, especially in maritime events and disasters, can be captured in order to have a more complete picture of drowning situations in the Philippines.

Similarly, investment in research on child drowning and its prevention in the Philippines is needed, including the role of determinants of health. A quality surveillance system for drowning incidents, such as ONEISS, will allow for detailed epidemiological studies to be undertaken, tracking trends over time, evaluating the impact of any prevention strategies that are enacted, and identifying emerging issues. Monitoring and evaluation of the implementation of, and progress against, the activities within the multisector action plan on drowning are also key. This will allow the relevance and effectiveness of the activities within the plan to be assessed, as well as guide the development of future iterations of the plan. Ensuring that the actions from these activities are specific, measurable, achievable, realistic, and timely (SMART) [63] will also help with ensure success.

4.7. Strengths and Limitations of this Study

This study represents the first of its kind, exploring child drowning in the Philippines and the development of the multisector action plan on drowning prevention. This study makes an important contribution to the literature regarding the role and consideration of determinants of health in preventing drowning and provides guidance to other nations on the development of a national water safety plan (referred to as a drowning prevention plan in this paper) as recommended by the WHO.

However, this study is not without limitation. The data on child drowning used in this study are modeled data sourced from the GBD Data Viz Hub. Limited variables are available for analysis using this data, which limits understanding of causal factors implicated in child drowning in the Philippines. This limitation represents a call to action for investment in and interrogation of national-level data on drowning (both fatal and non-fatal) in the Philippines, including the role of determinants of health, to better inform future prevention efforts. Secondly, analysis of the activities of the multisector action plan on drowning prevention with respect to relevance to child drowning and the importance of inclusion of determinants of health was conducted by consensus among the authors. Others performing these analyses may have a different interpretation.

5. Conclusions

Child drowning is a significant public health concern in the Philippines and a leading cause of child mortality. While there is a slight downward trend seen in the data on child drowning in the Philippines, there is much more to be done. The development of a multisector action plan on drowning prevention aims to guide all-age drowning prevention in the Philippines and includes several activities specifically targeting children. These activities, and work done to prevent drowning more generally, must consider upstream actions that take into consideration the determinants of health such as the role of education, the risks posed by urbanization, the importance of WASH, and safe water transportation. Children from high-risk groups such as low socio-economic families, rurally dwelling families, and ethnic minorities must be of specific focus. Enhancement of the national injury surveillance system, which includes drowning, is vital and should guide future research and implementation and evaluation of child drowning prevention strategies. It is hoped that the identification of and work to address these determinants will reduce drowning risk among children, and also the general population, and, therefore, save lives.

Author Contributions: Conceptualization, J.P.G., A.E.P. and R.C.F.; methodology, J.P.G., A.E.P. and R.C.F.; validation, A.E.P., R.C.F., J.P.G., L.L.C., M.R.S.Z.U., J.J.R.M., J.J.L.G., R.E.C.M., L.L.O. and L.L.C.; formal analysis, A.E.P., R.C.F. and J.P.G.; writing—original draft preparation, J.P.G., A.E.P. and R.C.F.; writing—review and editing, A.E.P., R.C.F., J.P.G., L.L.C., M.R.S.Z.U., J.J.R.M., J.J.L.G., L.L.O. and R.E.C.M.; visualization, A.E.P.; supervision, R.C.F.; funding acquisition, J.P.G., L.L.O. and L.L.C. All authors have read and agreed to the published version of the manuscript.

Funding: The "Development of the Multisector Action Plan on Drowning Prevention in the Philippines, 2016–2026" was supported by the World Health Organization. Project Title: Technical Assistance on Developing National Multisectoral Strategy on Drowning Prevention, WHO Registration: 2015/585544-0.

Institutional Review Board Statement: Ethical review and approval were waived for this study due to the use of publicly accessible, de-identified drowning data and the process of developing the multisector action plan on drowning being deemed to not require institutional ethics board approval.

Informed Consent Statement: Not applicable.

Data Availability Statement: Drowning data explored in this study is accessible via the Global Burden of Disease (GBD) Compare Data Viz Hub https://vizhub.healthdata.org/gbd-compare/.

Acknowledgments: The authors would like to acknowledge the representatives of various government and non-government organizations that contributed in developing the Multisector Action Plan on Drowning Prevention in the Philippines, 2016–2026.

Conflicts of Interest: J.J.L.G. and R.E.C.M. are employed by the WHO in the Philippines. The WHO funded the multisector action plan on drowning prevention project. The other authors declare no conflict of interest.

References

1. World Health Organization. *Global Report on Drowning: Preventing a Leading Killer 2014*; World Health Organization: Geneva, Switzerland, 2014.
2. Franklin, R.C.; Peden, A.E.; Hamilton, E.B.; Bisignano, C.; Castle, C.D.; Dingels, Z.V.; Hay, S.I.; Liu, Z.; Mokdad, A.H.; Roberts, N.L.S.; et al. The burden of unintentional drowning: Global, regional and national estimates of mortality from the Global Burden of Disease 2017. *Study* **2020**, *26*, 83–95. [CrossRef] [PubMed]
3. Peden, A.E.; Franklin, R.C.; Mahony, A.J.; Scarr, J.; Barnsley, P.D. Using a retrospective cross-sectional study to analyse unintentional fatal drowning in Australia: ICD-10 coding-based methodologies verses actual deaths. *BMJ Open* **2017**, *7*, e019407. [CrossRef] [PubMed]
4. Peden, M. *Drowning World Report on Child Injury Prevention 2008*; World Health Organization: Geneva, Switzerland, 2008; pp. 59–77.

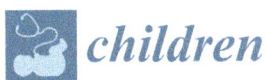

Article

Adolescent Water Safety Behaviors, Skills, Training and Their Association with Risk-Taking Behaviors and Risk and Protective Factors

Isabell Sakamoto [1,*], Sarah Stempski [1], Vijay Srinivasan [2], Tien Le [3], Elizabeth Bennett [1,2] and Linda Quan [1,4]

1. Seattle Children's Hospital, Seattle, WA 98105, USA; sarah.stempski@seattlechildrens.org (S.S.); tizbenharb1@gmail.com (E.B.); linda.quan@seattlechildrens.org (L.Q.)
2. School of Public Health, University of Washington, Seattle, WA 98195, USA; vs6563@uw.edu
3. School of Science, Technology, Engineering and Mathematics, University of Washington Bothell, Bothell, WA 98011, USA; tienle98@uw.edu
4. Harborview Injury Prevention Center, University of Washington School of Medicine, Seattle, WA 98195, USA
* Correspondence: isabell.sakamoto@seattlechildrens.org; Tel.: +1-206-987-6197

Received: 26 November 2020; Accepted: 15 December 2020; Published: 17 December 2020

Abstract: *Background*: Drowning remains the third leading cause of unintentional injury death for adolescents in the United States. *Aims:* This study described adolescent swimming lessons, behaviors (life jacket wear while boating) and comfort (swimming in deep water) and their association with protective and risk factors and risk-taking behaviors reported by Washington State students in Grades 8, 10, 12, primarily comprised of youth ages 13 to 18 years. *Methods*: This study used the 2014 Washington State Healthy Youth Survey (HYS), a publicly available dataset. *Results*: Most students reported having had swimming lessons, using life jackets, and comfort in deep water. Differences reflected racial, ethnic and socioeconomic disparities: being White or Caucasian, speaking English at home and higher maternal education. Lowest rates of comfort in deep water were among Hispanics or Latino/Latinas followed by Blacks or African Americans. Greater life jacket wear while boating was reported by females, those in lower grades and negatively associated with alcohol consumption, sexual activity and texting while driving. Having had swimming lessons was associated with fewer risk-taking behaviors. *Conclusions*: The HYS was useful to benchmark and identify factors associated with drowning risk among adolescents. It suggests a need to reframe approaches to promote water safety to adolescents and their families. Multivariate analysis of this data could identify the key determinants amongst the racial, ethnic, and socioeconomic disparities noted and provide stronger estimation of risk-taking and protective behaviors.

Keywords: injury prevention; drowning; water safety; adolescent; life jacket; swimming lessons; swimming ability; risk behaviors; protective factors

1. Introduction

Drowning is the third leading cause of injury death among adolescents 15 to 19 years in the United States (U.S.) [1]. From 2014 to 2018, the U.S. drowning death rate of adolescents ages 15 to 19 (1.1 per 100,000) was twice that of those ages 10 to 14 (0.5 per 100,000) [1]. Males were 5.3 times more likely to drown than females and Black or African American youth were 2.6 times more likely to drown compared to White or Caucasian youth [1]. In Washington State during this time period, the drowning death rate among those 15 to 19 (1.5) eclipsed other pediatric age groups [1]. Drownings in this age group in Washington State primarily involve swimming, playing, and boating in open water, like lakes or rivers [2].

High drowning rates among teens may be explained by their developmental stage. Adolescents are susceptible to peer pressure and engagement in risk-taking behaviors with a greater focus on rewards rather than costs and consequences [3]. In surveys and focus groups, adolescents have reported behaviors that put them at greater risk for drowning [4,5]. Risk factors such as neighborhood disorder may contribute to youth engaging in risk behaviors [6]. Fortunately, family and peer protective factors have proved effective in reducing risk behaviors like alcohol consumption at an early age [4]. It's unclear whether these behaviors are associated with other risk behaviors. Moreover, no studies have evaluated protective factors among adolescents with regards to drowning risk. To examine the risk and protective factors and risk-taking behaviors for drowning amongst Washington State adolescents, we evaluated self-reported risk and protective factors and risk-taking behaviors among adolescents taking the Washington Healthy Youth Survey (HYS). The HYS is an adapted version of the U.S. nationally administered Youth Risk Behavior Surveillance System (YRBSS), which is administered by the Centers for Disease Control and Prevention (CDC). Both the YRBSS and HYS include six categories of health-related behaviors that contribute to the leading causes of death and disability among youth and adults [7]:

- Behaviors that contribute to unintentional injuries and violence
- Sexual behaviors related to unintended pregnancy and sexually transmitted diseases, including HIV infection
- Alcohol and other drug use
- Tobacco use
- Unhealthy dietary behaviors
- Inadequate physical activity

We conducted a preliminary study to examine risk and protective associations between risk and protective factors and risk-taking behaviors with life jacket wear and formal swimming lesson participation amongst Washington State adolescents. Our goal was to use the HYS to better understand drowning risk and protection in the context of other adolescent risk-taking behaviors. Understanding those relationships could better identify which drowning factors might be associated with other general risk-taking and protective factors and better inform water safety promotion and drowning prevention interventions. Our objective was primarily to estimate the proportion of Washington youths who have had formal swimming lessons, wore life jackets (also known as personal flotation devices or PFDs) while boating and were comfortable in water over their head and characterize them. Additionally, we sought to evaluate risk-taking and protective factors around adolescents' wearing life jacket and having had swimming lessons.

2. Materials and Methods

2.1. Population

The HYS is conducted every two years to students in age Grades 6, 8, 10, or 12, primarily comprising youth ages 13 to 18 years [8]. All Washington public schools, except institutional or correctional schools, are invited to participate in the survey. Private schools can opt-in if they choose. Parents can decline their child's participation. Student participation is completely voluntary and anonymous.

Survey data from 2014 were used in analysis of this study. To create a statewide sample for 2014, Washington State schools were randomly selected by representative agencies of HYS administration (Washington State Department of Health; Office of the Superintendent of Public Instruction; Department of Social and Health Services' Division of Behavioral Health and Recovery; Liquor and Cannabis Board; and the contractor, Looking Glass Analytics, Inc., Olympia, Washington). A total of 35,262 students and 192 schools contributed to the statewide sample. All information obtained for this study is publicly available from www.AskHYS.net.

We limited this study to students in Grades 8, 10 and 12 surveyed in 2014 because these grades received the Forms with the questions of interest and this was the only year that all drowning prevention questions were included.

2.2. HYS Survey

The HYS surveys students for their health concerns, behaviors, school climate, quality of life, mental health, risk and protective factors and risk-taking behaviors. Behavioral questions addressed topics of alcohol, marijuana, tobacco, other drug use, sexual behaviors, and behaviors associated with intentional or unintentional injuries.

In this study, we focused on adolescents' responses to water safety questions regarding evidence-based drowning prevention interventions that decrease risk for drowning: a history of formal swimming lessons (i.e., lessons that were taught by a swim instructor are or that are received as part of another activity such as day care, school or camp) [9], use of life jackets [10,11] and swimming ability [5].

Students in grades 8, 10, and 12 completed Forms A/A-enhanced and B/B-enhanced [12]. Surveys were distributed randomly among students. This study assessed responses from B/B-enhanced only because it included all water safety questions. Form B consisted of 116 items derived primarily from the Youth Risk Behavior Survey and the Global Youth Tobacco Survey and included life jacket and swimming questions [12]. Form B-enhanced included six additional optional questions on sexual orientation, behavior and abuse. We assessed students who responded to the questions regarding swimming lessons (Q5), comfort swimming in deep water (Q6), and life jacket wear while boating (Q7). (Appendix A Table A1).

The HYS is available in English and Spanish. Spanish speaking students read a translated survey but respond on the English answer sheet to preserve anonymity [12]. Surveys were administered to all participating students in a single class period by a trained test administrator during the school day. Students completed surveys individually. Completed surveys were sealed and returned to Looking Glass Analytics by survey coordinators [12].

2.3. Variables

Demographic variables collected included student's gender, race and ethnicity, maternal education, language spoken at home, living situation, living arrangement due to finances, and grade level (details of these questions are located in Appendix A Table A1). We selected HYS questions regarding adolescent risk and protective factors and risk-taking behaviors by cross-referencing Jessor's Domains of Adolescent Risk Behavior and the 2014 HYS Questionnaire Form B/B Enhanced [13]. Categorization of chosen questions reflected the HYS framework for risk and protective factors and risk-taking behaviors [8]. HYS questions were reviewed for validity and reliability by experts in public health, injury prevention, and school health prior to inclusion in the administered survey [8]. The behaviors and factors chosen include unintentional injury behaviors (e.g., life jacket wear, exposure to swimming lessons), protective factors (e.g., eating dinner with family, having supportive adults), and risk-taking behaviors and risk factors (e.g., texting while driving, alcohol use, involvement in physical fighting) (Appendix A Table A1). These factors were not specifically related to water behavioral factors, but general lifestyle factors.

The three HYS survey questions related to drowning risks were: (Q5) have you ever taken formal swimming lessons?; (Q6) I am comfortable playing and swimming in water over my head; and (Q7) how often do you wear a life jacket when you're in a small boat like a canoe, raft, or small motorboat? (Appendix A Table A1). These questions were developed by drowning prevention experts at Seattle Children's Hospital, Washington State Department of Health and Public Health Seattle and King County and reviewed and approved by Washington State Department of Health prior to their inclusion in the HYS. Life jacket wear (Q7) was added to the HYS starting in 2002, and both swimming questions (Q5 and Q6) were added in 2014.

For this study, we used responses to the question about comfort in water (Q6) as a validated indicator of swim ability [5]. Taking formal swimming lessons and wearing life jackets are both validated drowning prevention indicators [9,10].

2.4. Analyses

This study used descriptive statistics. Respondents and their responses to each of the three water safety questions were analyzed separately.

The HYS includes the Q x Q analysis tool, publicly available through www.AskHYS.net [14]. This was used to analyze results for HYS questions by cross-tabulating two variables at a time for comparison. Collapsed versions for question responses were used for analysis by selecting the "collapsed" option in the query builder. Chi-Square tests were conducted using Microsoft Excel to estimate p-values to inform statistical significance of risk-taking behaviors, risk and protective factors associated with life jacket use and swimming lessons [15].

This Seattle Children's Institutional Review Board deemed that IRB review and approval was not required for this study due to its not involving human subjects.

3. Results

3.1. Descriptive Statistics

A total of 26,163 valid surveys from students in Grades 8, 10, and 12 across 167 schools were received for the 2014 HYS. Non-completion rates of Form B were 17% of Grade 8, 12% of Grade 10, and 9% of Grade 12; and for Form B-enhanced 17% of Grade 8, 14% of Grade 10, and 12% of Grade 12 [12]. A total of 10,456 students in these grades completed Form B or Form B-enhanced and responded to the question: "How often do you wear a life jacket when you're in a small boat like a canoe, raft, or small motorboat?" (Q7)—Of these, 2631 students indicated that they were never on a small boat; 13,120 students responded to the question: "Have you ever taken formal swimming lessons?" (Q5); and 13,095 students responded to the question: "I am comfortable playing and swimming in water over my head" (Q6).

The majority of students in Grade 8 were ages 13 to 14, Grade 10 were ages 15 to 16, and Grade 12 were ages 17 to 18 [8]. The majority of respondents identified as White or Caucasian; English was the primary language spoken in the majority of households (Table 1).

Table 1. Demographic characteristics of 2014 HYS Form B/Form B-enhanced Respondents' Life Jacket Wear While Boating, Exposure to Swimming Lessons and Comfort in Deep Water **.

Demographics	Life Jacket Wear When Boating		Had Swimming Lessons		Comfortable Swimming in Deep Water	
	Usually	Not Usually	Yes	No/Not Sure	Strongly Agree/Agree	Disagree/Strongly Disagree
Total N and Percentage	N = 5924 (56.7%)	N = 4532 (43.3%)	N = 7930 (60.4%)	N = 5190 (39.6%)	N = 11,351 (86.7%)	N = 1744 (13.3%)
Gender						
Male	2817 (47.6)	2423 (53.5)	3825 (48.3)	2658 (51.2)	5719 (50.5)	754 (43.4)
Female	3096 (52.3)	2104 (46.5)	4089 (51.3)	2526 (48.7)	5615 (49.5)	985 (56.6)
Race/Ethnicity						
American Indian or Alaskan Native	132 (2.2)	157 (3.5)	182 (2.2)	180 (3.3)	328 (2.9)	34 (2.0)
Asian or Asian American, Native Hawaiian or other Pacific Islander	701 (11.9)	373 (8.3)	876 (10.8)	612 (11.4)	1183 (10.5)	302 (17.5)
Black or African American	199 (3.4)	164 (3.6)	486 (6)	498 (9.3)	399 (3.5)	168 (9.7)
Hispanic or Latino/Latina	559 (9.5)	527 (11.7)	543 (6.7)	1213 (22.6)	1364 (12.1)	385 (22.3)
White or Caucasian	3447 (58.5)	2616 (58.0)	4910 (60.7)	2041 (38.0)	6390 (56.6)	555 (32.1)
More than one selected/other	852 (14.5)	668 (14.8)	1093 (13.5)	822 (15.3)	1623 (14.4)	285 (16.5)
Mother's Education						
High school or less	1366 (32.4)	1262 (29.9)	1591 (21.2)	2031 (40.2)	2961 (27.8)	660 (41.1)
More than high school	3420 (61.2)	2428 (57.5)	5080 (67.6)	1706 (33.8)	6191 (58.2)	589 (36.7)
Don't know/doesn't apply	801 (14.3)	532 (12.6)	846 (16.7)	1315 (26.0)	1492 (14.0)	358 (22.3)
Language spoken at home						
English	4805 (91.7)	3517 (81.7)	6581 (86.1)	3422 (70.1)	8925 (82.2)	1063 (64.6)
Spanish	312 (6.0)	339 (7.9)	298 (3.9)	823 (16.9)	830 (7.6)	287 (17.4)
Other	124 (2.4)	451 (10.5)	763 (10.0)	636 (13.0)	1103 (10.2)	296 (18.0)
Live with most of the time						
Parents/guardians	5337 (94.2)	3888 (90.7)	7181 (67.0)	1250 (71.6)	10,040 (92.9)	1488 (90.3)
Not parents/guardians	330 (5.8)	400 (9.3)	3541 (33.0)	496 (28.4)	764 (7.1)	159 (9.7)
Current living arrangements the result of losing home						
No/not sure	5394 (95.3)	3991 (93.9)	7209 (95.4)	3516 (91.4)	10,168 (94.9)	1500 (92.3)
Yes	265 (4.7)	260 (6.1)	344 (4.6)	330 (8.6)	547 (5.1)	126 (7.7)
Grade						
8	2711 (45.8)	1411 (31.1)	3161 (40.0)	2154 (41.5)	4621 (40.8)	674 (38.6)
10	1916 (32.3)	1686 (37.2)	2646 (33.4)	1816 (35.0)	3842 (33.8)	616 (35.4)
12	1297 (21.9)	1435 (31.7)	2123 (26.8)	1220 (23.5)	2888 (25.4)	454 (26.0)

** Column percentages.

Of the students who answered Q5, 60.4% reported having had formal swimming lessons. Male and female respondents had similar rates (59% versus 61.8%). Those who had had versus not had swimming lessons differed greatly in race and ethnicity, language spoken at home and maternal education. Most students who had had swimming lessons were White or Caucasian (60.7%) while those who had not had swimming lessons were non-White or Caucasian (62%), of which Hispanics or Latino/Latinas were the largest group. By race and ethnicity, White or Caucasian respondents had the highest rate (70.6%) of having had swimming lessons, followed by Asian or Asian Americans, Native Hawaiian or other Pacific Islander respondents (58.9%), and Black or African American respondents (49.4%). The lowest rate of swimming lessons (30.9%) was reported by Hispanic or Latino/Latina respondents. Among those whose mothers had had higher education, 75% of students had swimming lessons compared to 43.9% of students whose mothers had less education ($p < 0.01$). Similarly, among those whose primary language at home was English, 65.8% had had swimming lessons compared to only 26.6% of those whose primary language at home was Spanish.

Of the students who had been on small boats, 56.7% reported having worn life jackets. Females' wear rate was higher than males' (59% versus 53.8%). Notably, respondents who reported wearing life jackets versus not wearing them on small boats differed in language spoken at home and school grade. Those who reported life jacket wear while boating were more likely to speak English at home (56.6% versus 32.1%, $p < 0.01$). In contrast, respondents who did not wear life jackets were more likely to be Hispanic or Latino/Latina (11.7%) and not speak English at home (18.4%) (Table 1). Life jacket wear while boating decreased as grade level increased. Those who reported usually wearing a life jacket were less likely to be comfortable in water (87.7% versus 92.7%, $p < 0.01$).

Impressively, 86.7% of the responding students reported they were comfortable in deep water (Table 1). Respondents who were comfortable versus were not differed in race and ethnicity, maternal education, language spoken at home and grade in school. Those who were comfortable were mostly White or Caucasian (56.6%), spoke English at home (82.2%) and had higher maternal education (58.2%) (Table 1). When evaluated by race and ethnicity, almost all White or Caucasian respondents (92%) reported being comfortable in deep water; Black or African American respondents reported the lowest rates of comfort in deep water (70.3%). The percent comfortable swimming in deep water was highest among 8th graders and decreased with each subsequent grade.

3.2. Risk-Taking Behaviors and Risk Factors

Life jacket wear while boating was negatively associated with several risk-taking behaviors examined (Table 2). Students reporting life jacket wear while boating were less likely to have ever consumed alcohol than non-life jacket wearers (87.1% versus 69.9%, $p < 0.01$); less likely to have ever initiated alcohol use (60.3 versus 37.4%, $p < 0.01$) and if they had, were less likely to have initiated alcohol use at <14 years of age (23.4% versus 37.3%). They were also less likely to have ever had sexual intercourse (24.5% versus 32.2% $p < 0.01$) and less likely to be involved in physical fights (17.7% versus 28.9%, $p < 0.01$) compared to non-life jacket wearers. However, life jacket wearers were less likely to have used condoms than non-wearers (13.7% versus 21.7%, $p < 0.01$). Conversely, life jacket non-wear was associated with most risk-taking behaviors and risk factors examined, including alcohol use, sexual activity, involvement in a physical fight, and texting while driving.

Table 2. Risk-taking behaviors, risk and protective factors associated with life jacket use and swimming lessons **.

	Life Jacket Wearing When Boating		Swimming Lessons	
	Usually	Not Usually	Yes	No/Not Sure
Risk-Taking Behaviors				
Current alcohol consumption on any days *				
No days	5135 (87.1)	3149 (69.9)	1489 (18.8)	1017 (19.7)
Any days	763 (12.9)	1357 (30.1)	6412 (81.2)	4134 (80.3)
Number of lifetime sexual partners *,+				
Never	765 (69.9)	495 (54.2)	1683 (74.6)	984 (67.1)
1 to 3 people	279 (24.5)	294 (32.2)	433 (19.2)	361 (24.6)
4 or more	63 (5.5)	124 (13.6)	139 (6.2)	122 (8.3)
Condom usage during last sex act				
Yes	236 (13.7)	259 (21.7)	332 (14.7)	287 (19.5)
No	143 (8.3)	195 (16.4)	237 (10.5)	207 (14.1)
Never had sex	1340 (78.0)	739 (61.9)	1684 (74.7)	976 (66.4)
Was in a physical fight in the last 12 months *,+				
No times	4870 (82.3)	3215 (71.1)	1626 (20.5)	1293 (25.0)
Any times	1044 (17.7)	1306 (28.9)	6289 (79.5)	3882 (75.0)
Texted and drove in the past 30 days (among those who drove) *,+				
No days	1193 (67.4)	1061 (50.7)	2009 (59.6)	1206 (63.2)
Any days	576 (32.6)	1029 (49.3)	1360 (40.3)	701 (36.8)
Risk Factors				
Initiation of alcohol consumption +				
Never	3553 (60.3)	1680 (37.4)	4257 (53.8)	2507 (48.3)
13 or younger	1380 (23.4)	1678 (37.3)	2078 (26.3)	1696 (32.7)
14 or older	955 (16.2)	1138 (25.3)	1555 (19.7)	935 (18.0)
Protective Factors				
Eat dinner with family *,+				
Usually	3968 (68.1)	2551 (57.8)	5211 (67.0)	2739 (54.0)
Not usually	1859 (31.9)	1864 (42.2)	2565 (33.0)	2332 (46.0)
Getting along with parents *				
Completely true	2007 (36.5)	1158 (28.0)	2455 (33.2)	1522 (32.7)
Not completely true	3490 (63.5)	2982 (72.0)	4939 (66.8)	3130 (67.3)
Have adult support to turn to if feeling sad/hopeless *,+				
Yes	3362 (72.5)	2188 (63.0)	4307 (70.5)	2407 (60.1)
No	622 (13.4)	679 (19.6)	897 (14.7)	852 (21.3)
Not sure	654 (14.1)	605 (17.4)	908 (14.9)	744 (18.6)
Feel safe at school *,+				
Yes	5344 (90.3)	3816 (85.6)	7134 (90.1)	4358 (84.1)
No	576 (9.7)	640 (14.4)	786 (9.9)	821 (15.9)
Think about consequences before making a decision *,+				
Strongly agree/agree	4559 (87.4)	3228 (81.7)	6097 (86.2)	3568 (81.9)
Disagree/strongly disagree	655 (12.6)	723 (18.3)	976 (13.8)	788 (18.1)

** Column percentages. * $p < 0.01$ significant difference among life jacket wearers and non-wearers. + $p < 0.01$ significant difference among formal swimming lessons and no formal swimming lessons.

Students who had had swimming lessons and those who had not differed in prevalence of several risk-taking behaviors. Respondents who had swimming lessons were less likely to report initiation of alcohol at a young age (if at all), sexual activity, involvement in a physical fight, and texting while driving.

3.3. Protective Factors

Differences in the presence of protective factors were noted between life jacket wearers and non-wearers as well as those with and without a history of swimming lessons (Table 2).

All protective factors were significantly higher in those who wore life jackets and in those who had swimming lessons. Notably, respondents who reported wearing a life jacket when in a small boat were significantly more likely to usually have had dinner with their family than not (68.1% versus, 57.8%, $p < 0.01$). Similarly, those who had swimming lessons versus not were more likely to usually have had dinner with their family (67.0% versus 54.0%, $p < 0.01$). They were more likely to have adult support (70.5% versus 60.1%, $p < 0.01$), feel safe at school (90.1% versus 84.1%, $p < 0.01$), and think about consequences before making decisions (86.2% versus 81.9%, $p < 0.01$).

Those who had had swimming lessons were much more likely to be comfortable swimming in deep water relative to those who had not or were unsure (92.6% versus 77.6%, $p < 0.01$). While large percentages of both life jacket wearers and non-wearers were comfortable in deep water, those comfortable in deep water were less likely to wear a life jacket than to wear one (87.7% versus 92.7%, $p < 0.01$).

4. Discussion

This evaluation of a large number of teenage students across Washington State provided estimates of adolescents' life jacket wear, swimming lessons history and swimming ability. It demonstrated racial, ethnic and socioeconomic disparities and possibly underlying behavioral patterns that may underlie the differences.

The HYS can be useful as a surveillance tool to track life jacket wear, swimming lessons and swimming ability among adolescents—markers that have not previously been widely assessed. The reported 56% life jacket wear correlates well with observational studies of life jacket use among boaters [16]. The self-reported swimming lesson rate of 60% is the first estimate available for this age group but cannot be corroborated since swim programs do not report student enrollment numbers. Importantly, in this study, males and females reported similar rates of formal swimming lessons. Thus, disparities in swimming lessons cannot explain the marked disparity seen in male versus female fatal drowning rates where in the United States, between 2014 and 2018, the male death rate for unintentional drownings was 1.63 while the female death rate was 0.21 [1].

That 87% of students felt comfortable in water over their heads was surprising. Those comfortable swimming in deep water were more likely to have had swimming lessons and less likely to wear a life jacket. We used respondents' reports of being comfortable in water as a proxy for their swim ability based on a prospective study of school age students' estimation of their swim ability; being a "good swimmer" or "comfortable in deep water" correlated with the ability to pass a swim test at a public pool [5]. However, that validation study primarily involved school age youth of families with high income levels and few older adolescents. Importantly, surveys of older adolescent New Zealand males suggested that they overestimated their swim abilities [17]. Teens may overestimate their swim skills and abilities and underestimate water hazards—both of which increase their risk for drowning—due to their impulsive tendencies, lack of swimming experience, and peer pressures [18]. Additionally, others have reported that swimming ability is associated with lower life jacket wear [19].

This large cross-sectional study is the first to confirm race-based and socioeconomic differences associated with both swimming lesson history and swim ability among teenage students across a state. White or Caucasian versus non-White or Caucasian race/ethnicities and higher versus lower level of maternal education, the proxy for socioeconomic status, were inversely related to both swim history and swim ability. Previous surveys in the U.S., using multivariate methods, have shown racial and ethnic differences in swim competencies with Black or African American teens reporting lower swim abilities than White or Caucasian teens [20,21]. However, these studies addressed only large urban populations, especially inner-city children. A national survey of New Zealand high schoolers demonstrated racial and ethnic differences in swim competencies [22]. Like this study, it did not identify whether race or income level were independent predictors of swim competency.

A study of high school students in Turkey identified a significant relationship between adolescent rates of accidental injuries during school and their parents' education level similar to our findings [23]. The same study suggested the benefit of school and parental supports and policies for preventing injuries in adolescents [23]. In one U.S. study, youths' swim ability was better if parents could swim and encouraged them to swim [21]. In Thailand, using multiple logistic regression, swim ability was associated with income level, formal swimming lessons and guardian's swim ability [24]. Thus, families and schools may provide protective factors to prevent drowning. One next step in water safety promotion could be to encourage protective factors, like prosocial involvement and family involvement, to potentially reduce engagement in risk-taking behaviors and thus reduce drowning risk [25].

These findings also showed a consistent association between language spoken at home and responses to all three water safety behaviors and skills. Language spoken at home is a proxy for immigrant status, a variable rarely collected. Many countries have reported increased drowning risk among their immigrant populations [26]. In fact, Canada has focused its drowning prevention program on its "new Canadians" which includes a linguistic approach [27,28]. Water safety education programs must include input from culturally diverse and immigrant populations throughout program development and implementation and provide information for parents in languages other than English. Furthermore, it's essential that water safety programs recruit and retain lifeguards, swimming instructors, program administrators, and educators that reflect the communities that they aim to reach [26,28].

The results of this preliminary study support the usefulness of the HYS to explore the relationship of other adolescent behaviors and drowning risks. The HYS provided a unique opportunity to evaluate adolescents' water safety skills, behaviors and comfort in the context of risk-taking and risk and protective factors. The associations between risk-taking behaviors with life jacket wear and swimming lessons may imply that youth who don't wear life jackets or have formal swimming lessons are at greater risk for other adverse health-related conditions and events, like drowning.

We found that teenagers who wore a life jacket or had formal swimming lessons also experienced more positive familial and school relationships compared to those who did not wear a life jacket and did not have swimming lessons. Thinking about consequences before making a decision is one of 20 internal assets within the evidence-based Developmental Assets Framework [29]. One of their social competencies is planning and decision making indicating that a young person knows how to plan ahead and make choices. Drowning prevention recommendations could be included as part of skills training for adolescents related to decision making and risk reduction. Participation in swimming lessons may contribute to behavioral protective factors like critical thinking before making decisions. Programs should consider protective factors in the development of water safety and drowning prevention interventions and messaging as an approach to mitigate known risk factors for drowning [26]. Life jacket use and ability to swim, along with other water safety skills are considered core components of water competency [30]. Considering risk and protective factors and risk-taking behaviors within the context of water competency could be useful.

This study suggests a need to reframe how water safety is promoted to adolescents. One systematic review of multiple health risk behaviors (MHRBs) amongst adolescents presents the effectiveness of multiple health risk interventions—particularly in schools—for health-risk behaviors [31]. Incorporating drowning prevention as a component of widespread adolescent prevention programs in schools may be ideal for student participation and engagement in water safety education, and reinforcement of positive social norms, like life jacket wear, between peers and teachers [31].

Finally, this study identified a role of socioeconomic as well as cultural, language and racial differences in life jacket wear while boating and exposure to swimming lessons among adolescents. Students who wore life jackets and those who had had swimming lessons were mostly White or Caucasian and primarily spoke English at home. Conversely, life jacket non-wear was associated with being male and having low maternal education/lower income. Racial and ethnic differences were most marked between respondents who had swimming lessons versus not. White or Caucasian students were far more likely and Hispanic or Latino/Latina students least likely to have had swimming lessons compared to any other race studied. These differences underscore the need to provide access to swimming lessons among non-White or Caucasian, immigrant and lower income communities. Swimming programs should include organizations that reflect and serve culturally diverse communities to promote inclusivity and help reduce racial, ethnic and socioeconomic disparities in adolescent water safety behaviors and skills [25].

4.1. Limitations

This study has five limitations. First, the population studied did not represent all adolescents since it excluded teens who had dropped out of school and may not have included a representative sample of adolescents who attended private schools. Second, students with limited reading proficiency or those who spoke a language other than English or Spanish may not have had the same opportunity to complete the survey. Third, findings may not be generalizable as Washington State has had a strong drowning prevention focus that promoted life jacket use for over twenty years. Fourth, the self-report data may be influenced by memory, social desirability, reading ability, and developmental changes and tend to be overestimated [12]. However, the correlation between reported and observed life jacket use while boating rate was reaffirming [16]. This study was cross-sectional so potential correlations can only be inferred.

Finally, this study was unable to evaluate the associations using individual based responses which would allow complex univariate or multivariate analysis. The HYS dataset is publicly available but restricted in the amount and type of data available. To perform further analyses including multivariate analyses required access to individuals' data which required review and approval by the Washington State Department of Health and Institutional Review Board. Due to demands of the COVID-19 pandemic, limited state resources precluded review by both entities in our allotted time frame.

4.2. Future Research

Future studies could explore:

- How exposure to protective factors influences adolescents' attitudes and behaviors towards life jacket use and adoption of water competencies such as learning CPR and self-awareness of swimming limitation [30,32].
- The role of access to swimming lessons versus cultural attitudes in increasing swim comfort amongst racial/ethnic groups [25].
- Family and community factors in providing youth with swimming lessons and the scale of this impact.
- The relationship between having had formal swimming lessons and engaging in high-risk behavior.
- Differences between urban, suburban and rural youth.

5. Conclusions

This study demonstrated the usefulness of the Washington State HYS dataset to evaluate drowning risk and protection in the context of other adolescent risk-taking behaviors. The findings provide surveillance data but also new insights into drowning injury. They suggest the need to reframe our thinking and approach to promoting water safety to adolescents and their families. Findings align with previous studies' that youth experiencing low socioeconomic status and racial and ethnic disparities—specifically Black and African American and Hispanic and Latino or Latina—are at a significant disadvantage concerning swimming ability and water safety behaviors [20,21,33]. This study suggests identifying risk-taking adolescents as being at greater risk for drowning, identifying non-White or Caucasian and low income communities for improved access to swimming lessons, and a more holistic approach to life jacket use in teens by addressing risk-taking behaviors, risk and protective factors and emphasizing that swim ability does not mean that a life jacket is needed less often. Further evaluation of associations between risk-taking behaviors and life jacket usage may help identify psychosocial predecessors of risk-taking behaviors.

Author Contributions: Conceptualization, V.S., T.L., E.B. and L.Q.; data curation, I.S., S.S., V.S. and T.L.; formal analysis, S.S.; supervision, E.B. and L.Q.; writing—original draft, I.S., S.S., V.S. and T.L.; writing—review and editing, I.S., S.S., T.L., E.B. and L.Q. All authors have read and agreed to the published version of the manuscript.

Funding: This study was funded by Seattle Children's Hospital Community Health and Benefit Department, with in-kind support from Harborview Injury Prevention and Research Center INSIGHT Program.

Acknowledgments: We would like to acknowledge the INSIGHT Program, Emma Gause, Brianna Mills, and Erin Morgan, Harborview Injury Prevention and Research Center for their input to the study; Anar Shaw and Will Hitchcock, Washington State Department of Health; Molly Adrian, Seattle Children's Hospital Research Institute; William Koon, University of New South Wales; and all the students who participated in the Healthy Youth Survey.

Conflicts of Interest: The authors declare no conflict of interest.

Ethics: The Seattle Children's Hospital Institutional Review Board (IRB) determined that review was not required for this study as the study was based on an anonymous public use data set with no identifiable information on the survey participants.

Appendix A

Table A1. Questions studied from 2014 Washington State Healthy Youth Survey Form B and Form B-enhanced.

Question	Response Options
Unintentional Injury Behaviors	
Q5. Have you ever taken formal swimming lessons?	(a) Yes, (b) no, (c) not sure
Q7. How often do you wear a life jacket when you're in a small boat like a canoe, raft, or small motorboat?	(a) Never go boating in a small boat, (b) never, (c) less than half the time, (d) about half the time, (e) more than half the time, (f) always
Protective Factors	
Q6. I am comfortable playing and swimming in water over my head.	(a) strongly agree, (b) agree, (c) disagree, (d) strongly disagree
Q12. I feel safe at my school.	(a) Definitely NOT true, (b) mostly not true, (c) mostly true, (d) definitely true
Q20. When you feel sad or hopeless, are there adults that you can turn to for help?	(a) I never feel sad or hopeless, (b) yes (c) no, (d) not sure
Q37. How often do you eat dinner with your family?	(a) never, (b) rarely (c) sometimes, (d) most of the time, (e) always
Q71. I feel I am getting along with my parents or guardians.	0 "not at all true" to 10 (completely true)
Q94c. When I make a decision, I think about what might happen afterward.	(a) Strongly, (b) agree, (c) agree, (d) disagree, (e) strongly disagree
Risk-taking Behaviors and Risk Factors	
Q8. During the past 30 days, how many days did you text or email while driving a car or other vehicle?	(a) I did not drive a car or other vehicle during the past 30 days, (b) 0 days, (c) 1 or 2 days, (d) 3 to 5 days, (e) 6 to 9 days, (f) 10 to 19 days, (g) 20 to 29 day, (h) all 30 days
Q11. During the past 12 months, how many times were you in a physical fight?	(a) 0 times, (b) 1 time, (c) 2–3 times, (d) 4–5 times, (e) 6 or more times
Q25. How old were you the first time you: Had more than a sip or two of beer, wine, or hard liquor (for example vodka, whiskey, or gin)?	(a) None, (b) 1–2 days, (c) 3–5 days, (d) 6–9 days, (e) 10 or more days
Q24. During the past 30 days, on how many days did you: Drink a glass, can or bottle of alcohol (beer, wine, wine coolers, hard liquor)?	(a) None, (b) 1–2 days, (c) 3–5 days, (d) 6–9 days, (e) 10 or more days
Q100. With how many people have you ever had sexual intercourse?	(a) I have never had sexual intercourse, (b)1 person, (c) 2 people, (d) 3 people, (e) 4 people, (f) 5 people, (g) 6 or more people
Q101. The last time you had sexual intercourse, did you or your partner use a condom?	(a) I have never had sexual intercourse., (b) yes, (c) no

References

1. National Center for Injury Prevention and Control. Web-Based Injury Statistics Query and Reporting System (WISQARS). Available online: www.cdc.gov/injury/wisqars (accessed on 1 July 2020).
2. Quan, L.; Pilkey, D.; Gomez, A.; Bennett, E. Analysis of paediatric drowning deaths in Washington State using the Child Death Review for Surveillance: What the CDR tells us and doesn't tell us about lethal drowning. *Inj. Prev.* **2011**, *17*, 28–33. [CrossRef] [PubMed]
3. Steinberg, L. Risk taking in adolescence: New perspectives from brain and behavioral science. *Curr. Dir. Psychol. Sci.* **2007**, *16*, 55–59. [CrossRef]
4. Quan, L.; Crispin, B.; Bennett, E.; Gomez, A. Beliefs and practices to prevent drowning among Vietnamese-American adolescents and parents. *Inj. Prev.* **2006**, *12*, 427–429. [CrossRef] [PubMed]
5. Mercado, M.; Quan, L.; Bennett, E.; Gilchrist, J.; Levy, B.; Robinson, C.; Wendorf, K.; Fife, M.; Stevens, M.; Lee, R. Can you really swim? Validation of self and parental reports of swim skill with an inwater swim test among children attending community pools in Washington State. *Inj. Prev.* **2016**, *22*, 253–260. [CrossRef] [PubMed]
6. Byrnes, H.; Miller, B.; Morrison, C.; Wiebe, D.; Woychik, M.; Wiehe, S. Association of environmental indicators with teen alcohol use and problem behavior: Teens' observations vs. objectively-measured indicators. *Health Place.* **2017**, *43*, 151–157. [CrossRef] [PubMed]
7. Washington State Healthy Youth Survey. Data Analysis & Technical Assistance Manual. Available online: https://www.askhys.net/Docs/Analysis%20Manual%20for%202014%20and%202016%208-30-16.pdf (accessed on 22 June 2020).
8. Healthy Youth Survey 2014 Report of Results. Available online: www.AskHYS.net (accessed on 6 October 2020).
9. Brenner, R.; Raneja, G.; Haynie, D.; Trumble, A.; Xian, C.; Klinger, R.; Klebanoff, M. Association between swimming lessons and drowning in childhood: A case-controlled study. *Arch Pediatr. Adoles. Med.* **2009**, *163*, 203–210. [CrossRef]
10. Cummings, P.; Mueller, B.; Quan, L. Association between wearing a personal floatation device and death by drowning among recreational boaters: A matched cohort analysis of United States Coast Guard data. *Inj. Prev.* **2011**, *17*, 156–159. [CrossRef]
11. Stempski, S.; Schiff, M.; Bennett, E.; Quan, L. A case-controlled study of boat-related injuries and fatalities in Washington State. *Inj. Prev.* **2014**, *20*, 232–237. [CrossRef]
12. Healthy Youth Survey 2014 Analytic Report. Washington State Department of Social and Health Services, Department of Health, Office of the Superintendent of Public Instruction, and Liquor and Cannabis Board. Available online: https://www.askhys.net/Docs/HYS%202014%20Analytic%20Report%20FINAL%204-5-2016.pdf (accessed on 17 September 2020).
13. Jessor, R. Risk behavior in adolesence: A psychological framework for understanding and action. *J. Adolesc. Health* **1991**, *12*, 597–605. [CrossRef]
14. Healthy Youth Survey. Q × Q Analysis. Available online: https://www.askhys.net/Analyzer (accessed on 6 July 2020).
15. Agresti, A. *An Introduction to Categorical Data Analysis*; John Wiley & Sons: Hoboken, NJ, USA, 2007.
16. Chung, C.; Quan, L.; Bennett, E.; Kernic, M.; Ebel, B. Informing policy on open water drowning prevention: An observational survey of life jacket use in Washington State. *Inj. Prev.* **2014**, 238–243. [CrossRef]
17. Moran, K. Will they sink or swim? New Zealand youth water safety knowledge and skills. *Int. J. Aquat. Res.* **2008**, *2*, 114–127. [CrossRef]
18. American Academy of Pediatrics. Water Safety for Teens. Available online: https://www.healthychildren.org/English/safety-prevention/at-play/Pages/Water-Safety-for-Older-Children.aspx (accessed on 11 December 2020).
19. Peden, A.; Demant, D.; Hagger, M.; Hamilton, K. Personal, social, and environmental factors associated with lifejacket wear in adults and children: A systematic literature review. *PLoS ONE* **2018**, *13*. [CrossRef] [PubMed]
20. Irwin, C.; Iriwn, R.; Ryan, T.; Drayer, J. Urban minority youth swimming (in)ability in the United States and associated demographic characteristics: Toward a drowning prevention plan. *Inj. Prev.* **2009**, *15*, 234–239. [CrossRef] [PubMed]

21. Pharr, J.; Irwin, C.; Layne, T.; Irwin, R. Predictors of swimming ability among children and adolescents in the United States. *Sports* **2018**, *6*, 17. [CrossRef]
22. Moran, K. Parents, pals, or pedagogues? How youth learn about water safety. *Int. J. Aquat. Res. Educ.* **2009**, *3*. [CrossRef]
23. Kılınç, E.; Gür, K. Behaviours of adolescents towards safety measures at school and in traffic and their health beliefs for injuries. *Int. J. Nurs. Pract.* **2020**, *26*. [CrossRef]
24. Laosee, O.; Gilchrist, J.; Khiewyoo, J.; Somrongthong, R.; Sitthi-amorn, C. Predictors of swimming skill of primary schools children in rural Thailand. *Int. J. Aquat. Res. Educ.* **2011**, *5*. [CrossRef]
25. Stempski, S.; Liu, L.; Grow, M.; Pomietto, M.; Chung, C.; Shumann, A.; Bennett, E. Everyone Swims: A community partnership and policy approach to address health disparities in drowning and obesity. *Health Educ. Behav.* **2015**, *42*, 106S–114S. [CrossRef]
26. Wilcox-Pidgeon, S.; Franklin, R.; Leggat, P.; Devine, S. Identifying a gap in drowning prevention: High-risk populations. *Inj. Prev.* **2020**, *26*, 279–288. [CrossRef]
27. Water Safety New Zealand Report on Drowning. 2011. Available online: Tcdn-flightdec.userfirst.co.nz/uploads/sites/watersafety/files/Drowning_Report/WSNZ_Drowning_Report_2011_FINAL.pdf (accessed on 14 November 2020).
28. Golob, M.; Giles, A.; Rich, K. Enhancing the relevance and effectiveness of water safety education for ethnic and racial minorities. *Int. J. Aquat. Res. Educ.* **2013**, *7*. [CrossRef]
29. Search Institute. Available online: www.search-institute.org (accessed on 23 November 2020).
30. Stallman, R.; Moran, K.; Quan, L.; Langendorfer, S. From swimming skill to water competence: Towards a more inclusive drowning prevention future. *Int. J. Aquat. Res. Educ.* **2017**, *10*. [CrossRef]
31. Hale, D.; Fitzgerald-Yau, N.; Viner, R. A systematic review of effective interventions for reducing multiple health risk behaviors in adolescence. *Am. J. Public Health* **2014**, *104*, e19–e41. [CrossRef] [PubMed]
32. Water Safety USA. Available online: https://www.watersafetyusa.org/ (accessed on 22 October 2020).
33. Irwin, R.; Drayer, J.; Ryan, T.; Southall, R. *Constraints Impacting Minority Swimming Participation*; The University of Memphis: Memphis, TN, USA, 2008.

Publisher's Note: MDPI stays neutral with regard to jurisdictional claims in published maps and institutional affiliations.

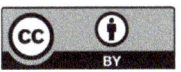

© 2020 by the authors. Licensee MDPI, Basel, Switzerland. This article is an open access article distributed under the terms and conditions of the Creative Commons Attribution (CC BY) license (http://creativecommons.org/licenses/by/4.0/).

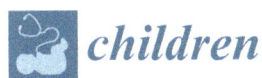

Article

Exploring the Impact of Remoteness and Socio-Economic Status on Child and Adolescent Injury-Related Mortality in Australia

Amy E. Peden [1,2,*] and Richard C. Franklin [2]

1. School of Population Health, UNSW Sydney, Kensington, NSW 2052, Australia
2. College of Public Health, Medical and Veterinary Sciences, James Cook University, Townsville, QLD 4811, Australia; richard.franklin@jcu.edu.au
* Correspondence: a.peden@unsw.edu.au

Received: 26 November 2020; Accepted: 20 December 2020; Published: 24 December 2020

Abstract: Injuries are a leading cause of harm for children. This study explores the impact of determinants of health on children (0–19 years) injury-related mortality (namely remoteness and socio-economic disadvantage, calculated using the index of relative socio-economic advantage and disadvantage (IRSAD)). Cause of death data from the Australian Bureau of Statistics were sourced for children in Australia between 1 July 2007 to 30 June 2017. Fifteen injury categories (ICD-10-AM external cause codes) were used. Burden and trends by injury mechanism were explored. A total of 5153 children died; with road traffic incidents (3.39 per 100,000 population), intentional self-harm (2.46) and drowning (0.72) being the leading mechanisms. Female fatality rates in very remote areas (8.73) were nine times higher than in major cities (Relative Risk [RR] = 8.73; 95% Confidence Interval [95% CI]: 4.23–18.00). Fatality rates increased with remoteness; very remote areas recording an injury-related fatality rated six times (RR = 5.84; 95 %CI: 3.76–9.12) that of major city residents. Accidental poisoning and intentional self-harm fatalities were more likely in high IRSAD areas, while road traffic fatalities were more likely in low and mid socio-economic areas ($X^2 = 69.1$; $p < 0.001$). People residing in regional and remote areas and from low socio-economic backgrounds already face significant health and lifestyle challenges associated with disadvantage. It is time to invest in injury prevention interventions for these populations, as well as upstream policy strategies to minimize any further preventable loss of life.

Keywords: injury; child; adolescent; risk factor; rurality; socio-economic; determinants of health; road traffic injury; falls; poisoning; drowning; violence; self-harm; prevention; intervention; epidemiology

1. Introduction

Globally, injuries are a leading cause of mortality and morbidity for children and adolescents. In 2017, the Global Burden of Disease study estimated 4.48 million injury deaths globally, an increase of 5.3% since 1990 [1]. However, some progress is being made in reducing injury-related deaths, with both years of life lost and age-standardized mortality rates decreasing between 1990 and 2017 [1]. Injury-related morbidity is also a significant global concern. New cases of non-fatal injury are increasing, with 520 million cases recorded globally in 2017, while years lived with a disability also increased [1].

Understanding and preventing injuries is complex as they may be intentional or unintentional, be due to a range of mechanisms such as road transport, falls, drowning, burns, poisoning, interpersonal violence and suicide, impact all ages and require a range of strategies to prevent them from occurring [1–4]. As the risk factors and prevention strategies needed to address unintentional and intentional injuries often differ, there is a need for studies which explore the causes of injury by age groups.

Injury risk is impacted by external factors including determinants of health. Determinants of health, referred to as the causes of the causes [5], are the conditions in which people are born, grow, live, work and play which impact health [6]. Determinants which impact health, including injury risk, include socio-economic conditions, daily living conditions, education levels and individual health-related factors [7,8]. Addressing the determinants of health helps to prevent events from occurring [5]. Strategies to prevent injuries need to be designed to address injury risk using a range of strategies from downstream (individual level) to upstream (system level), otherwise they are likely to be ineffective, especially when used in isolation, and must address underlying determinants of health [9].

Geographical remoteness and socio-economic status are determinants which impact health, including injury [10,11]. Poorer health outcomes are seen in rural dwelling populations, with greater hospitalization rates and disease burden [12,13]. This increased injury risk in rural locations also goes hand in hand with socio-economic disadvantage [14], which has been identified as a factor impacting injury risk [15–18]. Effective injury prevention strategies must consider these (and other) determinants of health when identifying areas of need and designing interventions.

Children and adolescents experience significant fatal and non-fatal burden due to injuries [19] and are particularly vulnerable to harm due to drowning [2,20], falls [3,21] and road traffic injuries [4,22]. Reducing injury-related mortality and morbidity is vital in order for nations to meet child and adolescent health targets within the Sustainable Development Goals [23,24]. Reducing injury-related harm among children and adolescents represents the area where the greatest health gains can be made [25].

While fatal child injury rates are declining, there are clear variations based on socioeconomic inequalities [26]. Therefore, within an Australian context, this study aims to explore injury-related mortality among children and adolescents to identify the impact of determinants of health, specifically rurality and a composite measure of socio-economic advantage and disadvantage (Index of Relative Socio-economic Advantage and Disadvantage (IRSAD)) of residential location, with an aim to inform future prevention efforts.

2. Materials and Methods

This study reports a total population analysis of injury-related mortality among children and adolescents aged 0–19 years (henceforth referred to as children) in Australia between 1 January 2007 and 30 June 2017 (a period of 10 years), with a particular focus on determinants of health—namely remoteness and IRSAD of the child's residential location.

2.1. Data Source

Cause of Death Unit Record File data were sourced from the Australian Bureau of Statistics (ABS). Data are provided to approved applicants only, but similar publicly available data to the Cause of Death data release collated by the ABS annually are provided [27]. Variables made available for analysis were date of death, sex, age group, jurisdiction of death (Australian state or territory and statistical local area), International Classification of Disease (ICD)-10 cause of death code and statistical local area. A statistical local area is a geographical area as used by the ABS. This study specifically uses statistical area level 2 which represents a community that interacts together socially and economically [28].

2.2. Case Identification and Data Cleaning

All deaths that had a primary cause of death injury ICD-10-AM [29] code were selected; only cases where the incident occurred during the study period were included, people who were aged less than 20 years were included and those who resided in Australia (i.e., visitors to Australia were excluded). Prior to commencing data coding and analysis, a total of 75 cases were removed; being 54 overseas residents and 21 with unknown residence.

This study examines injury-related deaths that were registered and who died between 1 January 2007 and 31 December 2017; noting that particularly for 2017, this would represent an approximate under-numeration of 6% (this proportion is based on the proportion of people who died within a given year but whose death was not registered until the following year). This particularly impacts those deaths which occur later in the year i.e., November and December. As such, trends over time are explored on Australian financial years 1 July to 30 June, from 1 July 2007 to 30 June 2017.

2.3. Coding of Injury Mechanisms

Fifteen categories of injury mechanism were collated using the ICD-10 codes. Due to small numbers of cases, the mechanisms of 'overexertion, strenuous and repetitive movements' (X50) and 'contact with venomous animals and plants' (X20-29) were grouped into 'Other'. The coding structure for the categories is described in Table 1.

Table 1. Injury categories used in study and associated International Classification of Diseases (ICD)-10 codes.

Injury Mechanisms Category.	ICD-10 Code	Code Explanation
Road traffic and other land transport	V00–V09	Pedestrian injured in transport accident
	V10–V19	Pedal cycle rider injured in transport accident
	V20–V29	Motorcycle rider injured in transport accident
	V30–V39	Occupant of three-wheeled motor vehicle injured in transport accident
	V40–V49	Car occupant injured in transport accident
	V50–V59	Occupant of pick-up truck or van injured in transport accident
	V60–V69	Occupant of heavy transport vehicle injured in transport accident
	V70–79	Bus occupant injured in transport accident
	V80–89	Other land transport accidents
Water transport, air and space transport and other/unspecified	V90–94	Water transport accidents
	V95–V97	Air and space transport accidents
	V98–V99	Other and unspecified transport accidents
Falls	W00–W19	Slipping, tripping, stumbling and falls
Exposure to mechanical forces	W20–W49	Exposure to inanimate mechanical forces
	W50–W64	Exposure to animate mechanical forces
Drowning	W65–74	Accidental non-transport drowning and submersion
Other accidental threats to breathing	W75–W84	Other accidental threats to breathing
Electrocution, radiation and extreme temperature	W85–W99	Exposure to electrical current, radiation and extreme ambient air temperature and pressure
Burns	X00–X09	Exposure to smoke, fire and flames
	X10–X19	Contact with heat and hot substances
Forces of nature	X30–X39	Exposure to forces of nature
Accidental poisoning	X40–X49	Accidental poisoning by and exposure to noxious substances
Accidental exposure to other forces	X51–X59	Accidental exposure to other specified factors
Intentional self-harm	X60–X84	Intentional self-harm
Assault	X85–Y09	Assault
Undetermined intent	Y10–Y34	Event of undetermined intent
Other	X20–X29	Contact with venomous animals and plants
	X50	Overexertion and strenuous or repetitive movements
	Y35	Legal intervention and operations of war
	Y40–Y84	Complications of medical and surgical care
	Y85–Y89	Sequelae of external causes of morbidity and mortality

2.4. Coding of Determinants of Health

The impact of determinants of health on child injury risk was explored by remoteness and IRSAD. The remoteness of the child's residential location was calculated by matching the nine digit statistical local area (SLA) code to the corresponding Australian Standard Geographical Classification (ASGC) category (i.e., major cities, inner regional, outer regional, remote and very remote) [30].

The nine-digit SLA was also used to code the victim's residential location to the corresponding decile on the index of socio-economic advantage and disadvantage (IRSAD). IRSAD aligns the statistical local area with a decile ranking (1–10), with areas ranked 1 being the most disadvantaged. Victims' residential postcode current IRSAD was used as a proxy for their familial socio-economic status [31]. IRSAD includes 17 measures around: income, education, employment, car ownership, internet connection, disability, family structure and renting status [32], which are combined to produce 10 IRSAD deciles. The IRSAD deciles were coded to low (deciles 1–3), mid (deciles 4–7) and high (deciles 8–10) for ease of analysis. Data between 2006 and 2011 were coded to the socio-economic indexes for areas (SEIFA) classification in 2011 and data between 2012 and 2017 were coded to SEIFA 2016 [33].

2.5. Statistical Analysis

Temporal trends over time in fatal injury mechanism were explored using the linear calculation in Microsoft Excel 365 (Build: 13426.20274). Crude rates and relative risk (RR) with a 95% confidence interval (CI) were used to calculate the impact of remoteness of residential location on injury-related fatalities. Crude rates per 100,000 population were calculated for all children 0–19 years, by sex and by age group (i.e., 0–4 years, 5–9 years, 10–14 years and 15–19 years), using the population from June of each year [34]. Population data by ASGC classification are currently only available for years in which the national census has been conducted. Therefore, a two-year average for the population was calculated using census years (2011 [35] and 2016 [36]) and this was used with a 10-year average of the deaths to calculate crude annualized injury-related fatality rates for children per 100,000 population by ASGC remoteness classification. Rates were used to calculate relative risk (using a MedCalc calculator [37]), with a 95% confidence interval using the lowest rate as the control group.

Univariate and chi-square analyses (calculated in International Business Machines [IBM] Corporation Statistical Package for the Social Sciences [SPSS] V25 [38]) were used to explore the impact of IRSAD on injury-related fatalities. Population data by grouped IRSAD decile (low, mid, and high) and age group are not publicly available in Australia. Therefore, the proportional of the all-age population in Australia as at 2016 by grouped IRSAD decile was calculated and assumed to hold true for children aged 0–19 years across the study period. These proportions were used to calculate non-parametric chi-square tests of significance. A modified Bonferonni correction, as suggested by Keppel [39], was applied at the 0.05 level, where multiple categories within a variable have been analyzed.

2.6. Ethics Approval

This study received ethics approval from the James Cook University Human Research Ethics Committee (H6136). Due to ethical constraints associated with reporting small numbers, small cell counts less than five (and their associated percentages) are reported as not presented (NP).

3. Results

Across the study period, there were a total of 5153 children who died due to fatal injuries. As a rate per 100,000 population, injury-related mortality among 0–19-year-olds in Australia varied from a high of 10.80 in 2008-09 to a low of 7.26 in 2013–14. The temporal trend across the study period shows a decline (y = −0.3166x + 10.627; R^2 = 0.72) (Figure 1).

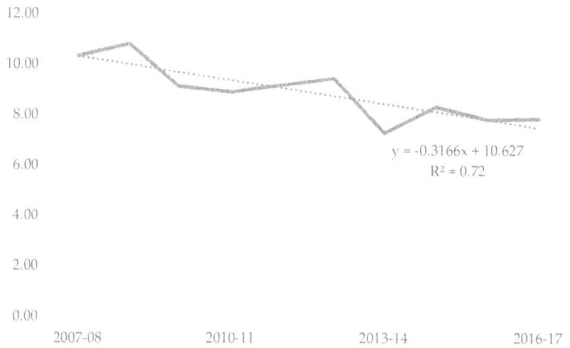

Figure 1. Crude rate per 100,000 of injury-related fatalities among children and adolescents 0–19 years, Australia 2007-08 to 2016-17.

The highest rates of fatal injury were seen in the 15–19 years age group with an average rate across the study period of 22.23 per 100,000, compared with the lowest rate of 2.63 per 100,000 among the 5–9 years age group. Crude injury-fatality rates are declining among 15–19-year-olds, with stagnant rates among 0–4-year-olds and 5–9-year-olds, with a slight upturn in rates among 10–14-year-olds (Figure 2).

Males accounted for 67.7% of all fatalities ($n = 3487$). Males were overrepresented in all age groups, rising from 59.1% of all injury-related fatalities in the 0–4 years age group, to 71.8% of all fatalities in the 15–19 years age group.

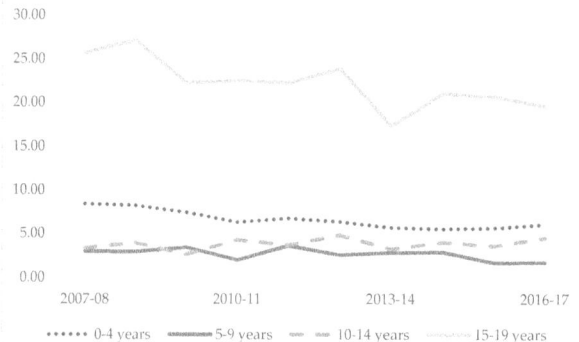

Figure 2. Crude rate per 100,000 of injury-related fatalities among children and adolescents 0–19 years, Australia 2007-08 to 2016-17.

Road traffic and other land transport incidents was the leading injury mechanism, accounting for 38.2% ($n = 1970$) of the overall injury-related fatality burden, followed by intentional self-harm ($n = 1432$; 27.8%) and drowning ($n = 419$; 8.1%). The overrepresentation of males was most pronounced in injury-related fatalities as a result of falls (82.6% male) and electrocution, radiation and extreme temperatures (80.0% male). When calculated as crude fatality rates, road traffic and other land transport incidents recorded a fatality rate of 3.39 per 100,000 population, compared to 2.46 for intentional self-harm and 0.72/100,000 population for drowning (Table 2).

Table 2. Incidence of injury-related fatality by mechanism, proportion of total and crude rate per 100,000 population among children and adolescents 0–19 years of age, Australia, 2007-08–2016-17.

Injury Mechanism	Incidence ($n =$)	Proportion of Total (%)	Crude Rate/100,000 Population
Total	5153	100.0	8.86
Road traffic and other land transport	1970	38.2	3.39
Water transport, air and space transport and other/unspecified	39	0.8	0.07
Falls	92	1.8	0.16
Exposure to mechanical forces	125	2.4	0.21
Drowning	419	8.1	0.72
Electrocution, radiation and extreme temperatures	15	0.3	0.03
Burns	112	2.2	0.19
Forces of nature	35	0.7	0.06
Accidental poisoning	167	3.2	0.29
Accidental exposure to other forces	39	0.8	0.07
Intentional self-harm	1432	27.8	2.46
Assault	292	5.7	0.50
Undetermined intent	144	2.8	0.25
Other accidental threats to breathing	228	4.4	0.39
Other	44	0.9	0.08

3.1. Impact of Social Determinants on Injury-Related Fatalities—Remoteness Classification

The rate of injury-related fatalities increased as remoteness increased. Major cities record a crude rate of 6.64 injury-related fatalities per 100,000 residents; rising to a rate of 38.90 per 100,000 residents in very remote areas. Very remote areas recorded injury-related fatalities at six times (RR = 5.84; CI: 3.76–9.12) the rate of major city residents (Table 3).

Table 3. Crude rate of injury-related fatality by remoteness classification, relative risk with 95% confidence interval, children and adolescents 0–19 years of age, Australia, 2007-08–2016-17.

Remoteness Classification	Proportional Population Distribution (%)	Crude Rate of Injury-Related Fatality/100,000 Population	Relative Risk (95% Confidence Interval)
Major Cities	69.9	6.64	1
Inner Regional	18.8	12.48	1.88 (1.52–2.31)
Outer Regional	9.0	15.41	2.32 (1.80–2.98)
Remote	1.4	25.75	3.88 (2.46–6.10)
Very Remote	1.0	38.90	5.86 (3.76–9.12)

Males recorded higher rates of fatal injury than females across all remoteness classifications, with the highest rates seen in very remote areas (12.52 for males compared to 9.79 for females). When compared to major cities, the relative risk of an injury-related fatality was six higher in very remote areas for males (RR = 5.62; CI: 3.20–9.87) and nine times higher for females (RR = 8.73; CI: 4.23–18.00). Rates of injury-related fatalities were highest for 15–19-year-olds across all remoteness classification, ranging from 17.11 fatalities per 100,000 residents in major cities, to a rate of 102.33 in very remote areas (Table 4).

Across the five remoteness classification categories, road traffic and other land transport incidents (2.45) and intentional self-harm (2.12) recorded the highest rates of fatal injury in areas classified as major cities. This pattern continued across all remoteness classifications, with the exception of very remote areas, where the rate of injury-related fatalities associated with intentional self-harm (16.97) overtook that of road traffic and other land transport (14.39). The highest RR of injury-related fatality was for electrocution, radiation and extreme temperatures, with an 18 times (RR = 18.24; CI: 0.02–18638.89) higher risk of dying from this injury mechanism in a very remote area than in a major city. (Table 5).

Table 4. Crude rate of injury-related fatality by remoteness classification, relative risk (RR) with 95% confidence interval (CI), children and adolescents 0–19 years of age, Australia, 2007-08–2016-17.

	Crude Rate of Injury-Related Fatality/100,000 Population								
	Major Cities	RR (95% CI)	Inner Regional	RR (95% CI)	Outer Regional	RR (95% CI)	Remote	RR (95% CI)	Very Remote	RR (95% CI)
				Sex						
Male	2.27	1	4.53	2.00 (1.55–2.57)	5.37	2.39 (1.76–3.24)	9.16	4.04 (2.35–6.97)	12.52	5.62 (3.20–9.87)
Female	1.08	1	1.93	1.77 (1.22–2.57)	2.58	2.36 (1.51–3.68)	4.40	4.00 (1.75–9.16)	9.79	8.73 (4.23–18.00)
				Age Group						
0–4 years	4.94	1	8.80	1.78 (1.08–2.93)	14.65	2.97 (1.74–5.06)	18.23	3.69 (1.33–10.21)	24.43	4.94 (1.72–14.20)
5–9 years	1.63	1	4.11	2.53 (1.17–5.44)	5.11	3.15 (1.28–7.74)	9.95	6.12 (1.45–25.77)	12.49	7.68 (1.71–34.55)
10–14 years	2.74	1	4.67	1.70 (0.87–3.33)	5.76	2.10 (0.94–4.71)	2.48	0.90 (0.26–3.17)	32.17	11.73 (4.14–33.26)
15–19 years	17.11	1	32.31	1.89 (1.46–2.45)	37.48	2.19 (1.58–3.03)	71.63	4.18 (2.29–7.64)	102.33	5.97 (3.28–10.88)

When compared to females, a proportionately higher number of males in the 0–4 years age group died from road transport and other land transport injuries in major cities (57.1%), rising to 79.3% for the 15–19 years age group in very remote areas. When compared to males, a proportionately higher number of females aged 10–14 years died due to road transport related injuries in very remote areas (62.5%). For intentional self-harm related fatalities, sex differences were most pronounced among 15–19-year-olds in inner regional areas, where males accounted for 73.1% of fatalities. Sex differences for drowning were most pronounced in major cities for the 15–19 years age group, with males accounting for 90.9% of all drowning-related fatalities.

Table 5. Crude rate per 100,000 population of injury-related fatality by mechanism and remoteness classification, relative risk (RR) and 95% confidence interval (CI), among children and adolescents 0–19 years of age, Australia, 2007-08–2016-17.

Injury Mechanism	Crude Rate of Injury-Related Fatality/100,000 Population									
	Major Cities	RR (95% CI)	Inner Regional	RR (95% CI)	Outer Regional	RR (95% CI)	Remote	RR (95% CI)	Very Remote	RR (95% CI)
Road traffic and other land transport	2.45	1	6.24	2.55 (1.86–3.48)	7.37	3.01 (2.06–4.38)	10.77	4.39 (2.17–8.89)	14.39	5.87 (2.83–12.18)
Water transport, air and space transport and other/unspecified	0.06	1	0.08	1.34 (0.12–14.92)	0.16	2.47 (0.20–30.66)	0.26	4.05 (0.04–385.50)	0.18	2.92 (0.01–1622.28)
Falls	0.15	1	0.18	1.20 (0.23–6.15)	0.25	1.70 (0.25–11.37)	0.64	4.30 (0.24–77.05)	0.37	2.47 (0.03–213.07)
Exposure to mechanical forces	0.14	1	0.35	2.46 (0.66–9.15)	0.49	3.45 (0.78–15.32)	1.15	8.15 (0.88–75.44)	2.03	14.33 (1.86–110.64)
Drowning	0.64	1	1.05	1.65 (0.82–3.35)	1.45	2.27 (1.00–5.15)	1.41	2.21 (0.33–14.93)	2.58	4.05 (0.74–22.22)
Electrocution, radiation and extreme temperatures	0.01	1	0.06	5.59 (0.10–305.20)	0.04	3.86 (0.02–828.20)	0.26	25.34 (0.12–5432.68)	0.18	18.24 (0.02–18638.89)
Burns	0.14	1	0.40	2.79 (0.79–9.90)	0.25	1.79 (0.27–12.09)	0.26	1.81 (0.02–156.60)	0.92	6.51 (0.36–117.53)
Forces of nature	0.05	1	0.10	1.95 (0.19–19.59)	0.10	3.68 (0.34–39.81)	0.13	2.41 (0.00–1373.41)	0.18	3.47 (0.01–1976.44)
Accidental poisoning	0.31	1	0.37	1.20 (0.38–3.76)	0.20	0.64 (0.08–4.91)	0.64	2.09 (0.12–35.44)	0.92	3.01 (0.18–51.00)
Accidental exposure to other forces	0.08	1	0.08	1.08 (0.10–11.30)	0.06	0.75 (0.02–31.72)	0.13	1.64 (0.00–887.94)	0.37	4.71 (0.05–432.97)
Intentional self-harm	2.12	1	3.22	1.52 (1.02–2.26)	4.32	2.04 (1.28–3.26)	7.69	3.63 (1.59–8.32)	16.97	8.02 (4.06–15.84)
Assault	0.50	1	0.41	0.83 (0.30–2.34)	0.96	1.92 (0.71–5.17)	1.03	2.06 (0.22–19.25)	1.11	2.22 (0.17–28.99)
Undetermined intent	0.20	1	0.51	2.58 (0.86–7.72)	0.43	2.18 (0.49–9.73)	0.38	1.95 (0.05–74.75)	0.55	2.81 (0.07–107.57)
Other accidental threats to breathing	0.34	1	0.47	1.40 (0.50–3.91)	0.72	2.15 (0.68–6.80)	1.92	5.72 (1.06–30.92)	1.29	3.84 (0.35–42.47)
Other	0.07	1	0.10	1.41 (0.71–2.83)	0.18	2.40 (1.14–5.07)	0.26	3.50 (0.83–14.65)	0.00	UTBC

UTBC = Unable to Be Calculated.

3.2. Impact of Social Determinants on Injury-Related Fatalities—Socio-Economic Classification

There was an annual average of 214 injury-related fatalities in areas classified as mid IRSAD decile, followed by 204 fatalities for low IRSAD decile residences. High IRSAD deciles recorded the lowest average, with 97 injury-related fatalities annually. Injury-related fatalities declined in all three IRSAD decile classifications across the study period, with the largest decrease occurring in the mid decile (y = −9.1273x + 264.4; R^2 = 0.6734). (Figure 3).

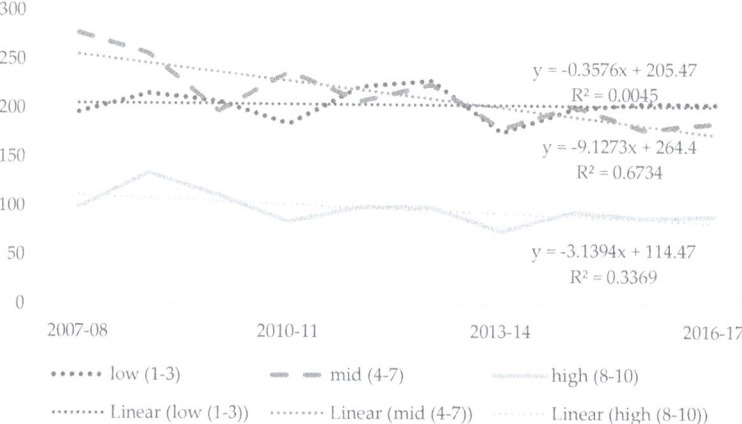

Figure 3. Injury-related fatalities among children and adolescents 0–19 years by index of relative socio-economic advantage and disadvantage (IRSAD) decile, Australia 2007-08 to 2016-17. Note: there were four cases with unknown IRSAD.

The highest proportion of injury-related fatalities occurred in areas classified as being mid IRSAD deciles (41.6%) and among males (67.7%). Males accounted for a higher proportion of injury-related fatalities than females across all IRSAD deciles. A higher proportion of female injury-related fatalities occurred among high IRSAD deciles (20.0%) than males (18.4%), however sex by IRSAD decile did not have a statistically significant impact on injury-related fatalities ($X^2 = 1.86$; $p = 0.395$). (Table 6)

Table 6. Injury-related fatalities by sex and index of relative socio-economic advantage and disadvantage decile (IRSAD), Australia, 2007-08 to 2016-17.

Sex	IRSAD Decile								X^2 (p Value)
	Total		Low (Deciles 1–3)		Mid (Deciles 4–7)		High (Deciles 8–10)		
	N	%	N	%	N	%	N	%	
Total	5149	100.0	2035	39.5	2142	41.6	972	18.9	
Male	3485	67.7	1387	39.8	1458	41.8	640	18.4	1.857 ($p = 0.395$)
Female	1664	32.3	648	38.9	684	41.1	332	20.0	

Note: excludes four cases with unknown IRSAD classification.

Across all age groups, the highest proportion of injury-related fatalities occurred in areas classified as low IRSAD, with the exception of the 15–19 years age group, where the highest proportion occurred in areas classified as mid IRSAD (36.9%). There was a statistically significant difference in injury-related fatalities for age group by IRSAD. Older children (15–19-year-olds) were more likely to die from injury-related incidents in areas classified as high IRSAD, whereas children (0–4 years) were more likely to die from injury-related incidents if residing in low IRSAD areas ($X^2 = 28.58$; $p < 0.001$) (Table 7).

Table 7. Injury-related fatalities by age group and index of relative socio-economic advantage and disadvantage decile (IRSAD), Australia, 2007/08 to 2016/17.

Age Group of Injury-Related Fatalities	IRSAD Decile								X^2 (p Value)
	Total		Low (Deciles 1–3)		Mid (Deciles 4–7)		High (Deciles 8–10)		
	N	%	N	%	N	%	N	%	
Total	5149	100.0	2035	39.5	2142	41.6	972	18.9	
0–4-year-olds	988	19.2	431 a	43.6	398 a,b	40.3	159 b	16.1	28.579 ($p < 0.001$)
5–9-year-olds	378	7.3	165 a	43.7	144 a	38.1	69 a	18.3	
10–14-year-olds	531	10.3	240 a	45.2	200 b	37.7	91 a,b	17.1	
15–19-year-olds	3252	63.2	1199 a	36.9	1400 b	43.1	653 b	20.1	

Note: excludes four cases with unknown IRSAD classification. Each subscript letter ($_{a,b}$) denotes a subset of IRSAD Grouped into Low Mid High categories whose column proportions do not differ significantly from each other at the 0.05 level using the Bonferroni adjustment (i.e., where there are two a's these are not statistically significant, where there is an a and b these are statistically significant).

Road traffic and other land transport was the leading mechanism of injury-related fatalities in areas classified as low IRSAD (38.9%) and mid IRSAD (40.7%). In areas classified as high IRSAD, intentional self-harm accounted for the highest proportion of injury-related deaths (32.4%). Statistically significant differences ($X^2 = 69.05$; $p < 0.001$) were found for proportion of injury mechanism by IRSAD for road traffic and other land transport (more likely in low and mid IRSAD deciles), accidental poisoning (high IRSAD), and intentional self-harm (low and mid IRSAD) (Table 8).

When exploring sex differences by injury mechanism, age and IRSAD decile, 15–19-year-old males accounted for a significantly higher proportion of drowning-related deaths in low (96.3% male), mid (89.2%) and high (90.9%) IRSAD deciles. Females aged 0–4 years old accounted for 71.4% of burn-related deaths in high IRSAD deciles. A higher proportion of males aged 15–19 years of age died from intentional self-harm in low IRSAD deciles (72.7% male) compared to mid (68.5% male) and high IRSAD deciles (66.1% male).

Table 8. Injury-related fatalities by age group and index of relative socio-economic advantage and disadvantage decile (IRSAD), Australia, 2007-08 to 2016-17.

Mechanism of Injury-Related Fatalities	Total		Low (Deciles 1–3)		Mid (Deciles 4–7)		High (Deciles 8–10)		X^2 (p Value)
	N	%	N	%	N	%	N	%	
Total	5149	100.0	2035	39.5	2142	41.6	972	18.9	-
Road traffic and other land transport	1970	38.3	791 a	40.2	871 a	44.2	308 b	15.6	
Water transport, air and space transport and other/unspecified	39	0.8	8 a	20.5	24 b	61.5	7 a,b	17.9	
Falls	92	1.8	29 a	31.5	40 a	43.5	23 a	25.0	
Exposure to mechanical forces	125	2.4	47 a	37.6	56 a	44.8	22 a	17.6	
Drowning	418	8.1	175 a	41.9	171 a	40.9	72 a	17.2	
Electrocution, radiation and extreme temperatures	15	0.3	5 a	33.3	6 a	40.0	NP a	NP	69.052 ($p < 0.001$)
Burns	111	2.2	38 a	34.2	55 a	49.5	18 a	16.2	
Forces of nature	35	0.7	12 a	34.3	16 a	45.7	7 a	20.0	
Accidental poisoning	167	3.2	52 a	31.1	72 a,b	43.1	43 b	25.7	
Accidental exposure to other forces	39	0.8	12 a	30.8	12 a	30.8	15 b	38.5	
Intentional self-harm	1431	27.8	555 a	38.8	561 a	39.2	315 b	22.0	
Assault	292	5.7	124 a	42.5	110 a	37.7	58 a	19.9	
Undetermined intent	143	2.8	65 a	45.5	54 a	37.8	24 a	16.8	
Other accidental threats to breathing	228	4.4	100 a	43.9	80 a	35.1	48 a	21.1	
Other	44	0.9	22 a	50.0	14 a	31.8	8 a	18.2	

Note: excludes four cases with unknown IRSAD classification. NP = Not Presented. Each subscript letter (a,b) denotes a subset of IRSAD Grouped into Low Mid High categories whose column proportions do not differ significantly from each other at the 0.05 level using the Bonferroni adjustment (i.e., where there are two a's these are not statistically significant, where there is an a and b these are statistically significant).

4. Discussion

Injury is a leading, yet preventable cause of death among children. This study has explored the impact of determinants of health, namely remoteness of residential location and IRSAD of residential location on injury-related fatalities among 0–19-year-olds in Australia. This study reports the injury-related fatalities of 5153 children aged 0–19 years, with the highest rates occurring among adolescents 15–19 years (22.23/100,000 population). The highest rates of injury-related fatalities being due to the mechanisms of road traffic and other land transport (3.39), intentional self-harm (2.46) and drowning (0.72). Rates of injury-related fatality increased as remoteness increased, with six times the risk of an injury-related fatality for children aged 0–19 years in very remote areas of Australia when compared to those residing in major cities. Males and 15–19-year-olds recorded the highest rates of injury-related fatality across all remoteness classifications and age bands, with the highest rate seen among 15–19-year-olds in very remote areas (a rate of 102.33/100,000 people).

Variations in fatal injury risk also exist based on the socio-economic advantage or disadvantage of where children live. While sex did not significantly impact injury-related fatalities when examined by IRSAD decile, significant differences were seen by age band and injury mechanism. Fatal injury risk was most pronounced in low IRSAD areas for very young children (0–4 years of age) and in high IRSAD areas for 15–19-year-olds. Road transport and other land transport injury-related fatalities and intentional self-harm fatalities were significantly more likely in low and mid IRSAD deciles, while accidental poisoning-related fatalities were significantly more likely in high IRSAD deciles. We now focus our discussion on the three leading injury mechanisms identified in the study being road traffic and other land-based transport, intentional self-harm and drowning. We then look to the future with respect to preventative efforts, while also focusing on the opportunity that the new National Injury Prevention Plan provides.

Road traffic and other land-based transport incidents accounted for the largest number of fatalities (n = 1970, 38%) across the study period. High rates were seen across all remoteness classifications, with the fatality risk associated with this mechanism six times higher (RR = 5.87; CI: 2.83–12.18) in very remote areas when compared to major cities. Similarly, road traffic injuries were significantly more likely in areas classified as low (n = 791, 40%) and mid (n = 871, 42%) IRSAD deciles. Road surfaces are generally of poorer quality in regional and remote Australia [40], there is a greater diversity of vehicles on the road [41], lower populations see lower investment in vital transport-related infrastructure [42] and higher speeds and driver fatigue all contribute to high fatality rates on regional Australian roads [43]. This, combined with regional dwelling populations often having to travel longer distances by road to seek major services including medical care [44–46], leads to increased exposure and risk of injury and death. Investment in higher quality rural roads which allow for passing and accommodate the wider range of vehicles may be a strategy to reduce injury-related fatalities [43], while upstream, policy approaches, such as investing in more regionally based doctors and specialist services [46] may also be required.

Socio-economic status impacts the mode of transport used [47]. For residents of low-socio economic areas, the use of lower cost, older vehicles with poorer safety standards may be contributing to an increased risk of death [43]. Strategies to combat this may be policy approaches such as subsidies to improve vehicle quality and investment in improving infant restraint fitting and correct use [48]. Research also indicates that residents of low socio-economic areas have higher exposure to traffic [49] and see lower investment in transport-related infrastructure [50]. Similar to addressing road traffic-related mortality in geographically isolated areas, multi-faceted strategies will be needed to reduce injury risk. For children and adolescents who are too young to drive, such strategies must take a whole community level approach and or target parents and caregivers.

Intentional self-harm was the second leading cause of injury-related mortality among children in Australia across the study period, accounting for 28% of all deaths. Intentional self-harm recorded the highest fatality rate of any mechanism in very remote areas (16.97 per 100,000 residents), a rate that is eight times (RR = 8.02; CI: 4.06–15.84) that of the fatality rate in major cities. Adolescence is a period of high risk for suicide, due to multiple stressors, mood disorders and development phase [51,52]. Though legislation in Australia significantly limits firearm availability and familiarity among potential users, compared to firearm-heavy nations such as the United States [53], increased access to firearms in rural areas may be a contributing factor to increased risk of intentional self-harm-related death in remote areas of Australia [54,55].

Like most other injury mechanisms explored, this study identified that the risk of an intentional self-harm-related fatality was significantly higher for residents of low and mid IRSAD deciles. The published literature has also identified this increased intentional self-harm risk in areas of socio economic disadvantage [56,57]. Given the impact of broader social factors on risk of intentional self-harm, upstream social and economic approaches that seek to redress socio-economic disadvantage of children and adolescents in Australia are recommended, beyond the provision of mental health services [58].

This study found drowning to be the third leading cause of injury-related fatalities among children in Australia. Like other injury mechanisms, rates increased as remoteness increased, aside from a slightly higher rate in inner regional (1.45 per 100,000 residents) than outer regional (1.41), with a four times (RR = 4.05; CI: 0.74–22.22) greater risk of drowning in very remote areas than in major cities. Similarly, a higher proportion of drowning occur in areas of low and mid socio-economic status, with just 17.2% of drowning deaths occurring in high socio-economic areas. This is in keeping with other studies into drowning which have identified significantly higher rates of drowning as rurality increases [59,60] and in low socio-economic areas [61,62].

A range of upstream factors also impact drowning risk, with less pools, seasonal facilities and a lack of instructors impacting ability to learn to swim in regional and remote areas [59], and the limited provision of school-based lessons and the high cost of private lessons a barrier for low-socio economic families [63]. Unpatrolled inland waterways used for recreation [60] and higher rates of alcohol consumption combined with aquatic activity [64], are also factors increasing drowning risk in regional and remote areas. Social determinants, such as remoteness and socio-economic disadvantage, are important factors impacting drowning risk and must be considered by drowning prevention practitioners. Very few drowning prevention initiatives targeting regional and remote communities have been evaluated [59], providing meagre evidence to direct limited funding to the most effective strategies.

Greater investment is clearly needed in primary prevention measures to reduce injury-related mortality and morbidity in regional and remote Australia and among areas of socio-economic disadvantage [65]. This will require also addressing the determinants of health and taking a wider lens when developing prevention programs, including ensuring programs are piloted in rural areas, engaging with families through co-design [66] and investing in infrastructure in low socio-economic areas [67]. Primary prevention measures must however, go hand in hand with improved tertiary prevention strategies, such as community first aid and cardiopulmonary resuscitation (CPR) [68] and trauma care services [69,70].

The existence of the new National Injury Prevention Strategy 2020–2030 [71], which identifies the impact of determinants of health such as remoteness and socio-economic status in many of its priority populations and priority areas, may serve as a driver to generate policy change and increased investment in addressing groups at increased injury risk due to determinants of health.

Preventing injury-related harm is vital to the nation's addressing many of the child and adolescent health targets outlined in the Sustainable Development Goals [23,24]. More broadly, injury prevention efforts intersect many global agendas such as healthy aging, climate change, water safeguarding, urbanization and corporate social responsibility [24]. As part of the United Nations' Decade of Action to 2030, leveraging the broader impacts of, and intersections with, injury prevention may present opportunities for greater political commitment to tackling this preventable cause of mortality and morbidity. This study has identified opportunities for further research, in particular the need for greater implementation and evaluation of injury prevention interventions targeted at residents of regional and remote and low socio-economic areas of Australia across a range of injury mechanisms. Advocacy to encourage greater investment in injury prevention in these disadvantaged areas will be strengthened by the evidence to support the best return on investment.

Strengths and Limitations

This study adds to the limited literature exploring the impact of injury related fatality among children aged 0–19 years in Australia by determinants of health, namely remoteness and socio-economic status of residential location at a total population level. The study uses a nationally validated data source and is likely to have consistency and accuracy with respect to the identification of cause of death. Where population data were available, this study uses rates to explore risk of injury-related fatalities per 100,000 residents.

There are, however, some limitations associated with this study. This study explores fatalities only, and further research is needed to explore the full burden of injury-related morbidity. Population data by IRSAD decile are not publicly available in Australia and therefore we were unable to calculate fatality rates by IRSAD. Assumption made regarding population distribution across the all-age population grouped IRSAD deciles holding true for children aged 0–19 years may not be correct. As such, the chi square tests of significance should be interpreted with caution. As remoteness and IRSAD are calculated at the statistical local area level, this limits any individual advantage or disadvantage which may occur within a statistical local area. For example, in an area considered to be low IRSAD, it is possible that there are households which would be considered high within the IRSAD classification. With respect to remoteness, some of the statistical areas are quite large, potentially spanning several remoteness classifications, however in this study, they have been assigned to a single remoteness classification.

5. Conclusions

This study has explored the impact of determinants of health, namely the geographical remoteness of residence and socio-economic status of residential area on injury-related fatalities among children aged 0–19 years in Australia. This study identified road traffic and other land transport injuries, intentional self-harm and drowning to be the three leading causes of death, with fatality rates increasing as remoteness increased. For most injury mechanisms examined that there was a disproportionate burden among low and middle IRSAD deciles except for intentional self-harm and accidental poisoning related deaths, which were significantly higher in high IRSAD areas. The findings of this study suggest injury prevention strategies for young people in Australia should consider these determinants of health. People residing in regional and remote areas and from low socio-economic backgrounds already face significant health and lifestyle challenges associated with disadvantage. It is time to invest in these populations to minimize any further preventable loss of life.

Author Contributions: Conceptualization, A.E.P. and R.C.F.; methodology, A.E.P. and R.C.F.; formal analysis, A.E.P. and R.C.F.; data curation, R.C.F.; writing—original draft preparation, A.E.P.; writing—review and editing, A.E.P. and R.C.F.; visualization, A.E.P. All authors have read and agreed to the published version of the manuscript.

Funding: This research received no external funding.

Institutional Review Board Statement: This study was conducted according to the guidelines of the Declaration of Helsinki, and approved by the Human Research Ethics Committee of James Cook University (H6136).

Informed Consent Statement: Informed consent was not able to be obtained as subjects are deceased.

Data Availability Statement: Agreements in place for use of data in this study place restrictions on the public storage of such data. Those interested in gaining access to the data used in this study, should contact the Australian Bureau of Statistics via email: client.services@abs.gov.au.

Conflicts of Interest: The authors declare no conflict of interest.

References

1. James, S.L.; Castle, C.D.; Dingels, Z.V.; Fox, J.T.; Hamilton, E.B.; Liu, Z.; Roberts, N.L.S.; Sylte, D.O.; Henry, N.J.; LeGrand, K.E.; et al. Global injury morbidity and mortality from 1990 to 2017: Results from the Global Burden of Disease Study 2017. *Inj. Prev.* **2020**, *26* (Suppl. 1), i96–i114. [CrossRef] [PubMed]
2. Franklin, R.C.; Peden, A.E.; Hamilton, E.B.; Bisignano, C.; Castle, C.D.; Dingels, Z.V.; Hay, S.I.; Liu, Z.; Mokdad, A.H.; Roberts, N.L.S.; et al. The burden of unintentional drowning: Global, regional and national estimates of mortality from the Global Burden of Disease 2017 Study. *Inj. Prev.* **2020**. [CrossRef]
3. James, S.L.; Lucchesi, L.R.; Bisignano, C.; Castle, C.D.; Dingels, Z.V.; Fox, J.T.; Hamilton, E.B.; Henry, N.J.; Krohn, K.J.; Liu, Z.; et al. The global burden of falls: Global, regional and national estimates of morbidity and mortality from the Global Burden of Disease Study 2017. *Inj. Prev.* **2020**, *26* (Suppl. 1), i3–i11. [CrossRef] [PubMed]
4. James, S.L.; Lucchesi, L.R.; Bisignano, C.; Castle, C.D.; Dingels, Z.V.; Fox, J.T.; Hamilton, E.B.; Liu, Z.; McCracken, D.; Nixon, M.; et al. Morbidity and mortality from road injuries: Results from the Global Burden of Disease Study 2017. *Inj. Prev.* **2020**, *26* (Suppl. 1), i46–i56. [CrossRef] [PubMed]
5. Braveman, P.; Gottlieb, L. The Social Determinants of Health: It's Time to Consider the Causes of the Causes. *Public Health Rep.* **2014**, *129* (Suppl. 2), 19–31. [CrossRef]

6. Marmot, M.; Friel, S.; Bell, R.; Houweling, T.A.J.; Taylor, S.; Commission on Social Determinants of Health. Closing the gap in a generation: Health equity through action on the social determinants of health. *Lancet* **2008**, *372*, 1661–1669. [CrossRef]
7. Laflamme, L. Explaining socio-economic differences in injury risks. *Inj. Control Saf. Promot.* **2001**, *8*, 149–153. [CrossRef]
8. Pickett, W.; Molcho, M.; Simpson, K.; Janssen, I.; Kuntsche, E.; Mazur, J.; Harel, Y.; Boyce, W.F. Cross national study of injury and social determinants in adolescents. *Inj. Prev.* **2005**, *11*, 213–218. [CrossRef]
9. Cenderadewi, M.; Franklin, R.C.; Devine, S. Socio-Ecological Nature of Drowning in Low-and Middle-Income Countries: A Review to Inform Health Promotion Approaches. *Int. J. Aquat. Res. Educ.* **2020**, *12*, 6. [CrossRef]
10. Mitchell, R.J.; Chong, S. Comparison of injury-related hospitalised morbidity and mortality in urban and rural areas in Australia. *Rural Remote Health* **2010**, *10*, 1326.
11. Coben, J.H.; Tiesman, H.M.; Bossarte, R.M.; Furbee, P.M. Rural–Urban Differences in Injury Hospitalizations in the U.S., 2004. *Am. J. Prev. Med.* **2009**, *36*, 49–55.
12. Strong, K. *Health in Rural and Remote Australia: The First Report of the Australian institute of Health and Welfare on Rural Health*; Australian Institute of Health and Welfare: Canberra, Australia, 1998.
13. Ziersch, A.; Baum, F.; Darmawan, I.G.N.; Kavanagh, A.; Bentley, R. Social capital and health in rural and urban communities in South Australia. *Aust. N. Z. J. Public Health* **2009**, *33*, 7–16. [CrossRef] [PubMed]
14. Larson, A. Rural health's demographic destiny. *Rural Remote Health* **2006**, *6*, 551. [PubMed]
15. Simpson, K.; Janssen, I.; Craig, W.M.; Pickett, W. Multilevel analysis of associations between socioeconomic status and injury among Canadian adolescents. *J. Epidemiol. Community Health* **2005**, *59*, 1072–1077. [CrossRef] [PubMed]
16. Birken, C.S.; MacArthur, C. Socioeconomic status and injury risk in children. *Paediatr. Child Health* **2004**, *9*, 323–325. [CrossRef]
17. Cubbin, C.; LeClere, F.B.; Smith, G.S. Socioeconomic status and injury mortality: Individual and neighbourhood determinants. *J. Epidemiol. Community Health* **2000**, *54*, 517–524. [CrossRef]
18. Cubbin, C.; LeClere, F.B.; Smith, G.S. Socioeconomic status and the occurrence of fatal and nonfatal injury in the United States. *Am. J. Public Health* **2000**, *90*, 70–77.
19. Peden, M.M. *World Report on Child Injury Prevention—UNICEF*; World Health Organization: Geneva, Switzerland, 2008.
20. Peden, A.E.; Franklin, R.C.; Clemens, T. Can child drowning be eradicated? A compelling case for continued investment in prevention. *Acta Paediatr.* **2020**, *0*, 1–8. [CrossRef]
21. Khambalia, A.; Joshi, P.; Brussoni, M.; Raina, P.; Morrongiello, B.; MacArthur, C. Risk factors for unintentional injuries due to falls in children aged 0–6 years: A systematic review. *Inj. Prev.* **2006**, *12*, 378–381. [CrossRef]
22. Sonkin, B.; Edwards, P.; Roberts, I.; Green, J. Walking, Cycling and Transport Safety: An Analysis of Child Road Deaths. *J. R. Soc. Med.* **2006**, *99*, 402–405. [CrossRef]
23. United Nations. Sustainable Development Goals Knowledge Platform—Sustainable Development Goal 3 2020. Available online: https://sustainabledevelopment.un.org/sdg3 (accessed on 7 July 2020).
24. Ma, T.; Peden, A.E.; Peden, M.; Hyder, A.; Jagnoor, J.; Duan, L.; Brown, J.; Passmore, J.; Clapham, K.; Tian, M.; et al. Out of the silos: Embedding injury prevention into the Sustainable Development Goals. *Inj. Prev.* **2020**. [CrossRef] [PubMed]
25. Harvey, A. Injury Prevention and the Attainment of Child and Adolescent Health. *Bull. World Health Organ.* **2009**, *87*, 390–394. [CrossRef] [PubMed]
26. Roberts, I.; Power, C. Does the decline in child injury mortality vary by social class? A comparison of class specific mortality in 1981 and 1991. *BMJ* **1996**, *313*, 784–786. [CrossRef] [PubMed]
27. Australian Bureau of Statistics. *Underlying causes of death (Australia) 2018*; Australian Bureau of Statistics: Canberra, Australia, 2019.
28. Australian Bureau of Statistics. Main Structure and Greater Capital City Statistical Areas. In *1270.0.55.001—Australian Statistical Geography Standard (ASGS)*; Australian Bureau of Statistics: Canberra, Australia, 2016; Volume 1. Available online: https://www.abs.gov.au/ausstats/abs@.nsf/Lookup/by%20Subject/

1270.0.55.001~{}July%202016~{}Main%20Features~{}Statistical%20Area%20Level%202%20(SA2)~{}10014 (accessed on 7 July 2020).

29. National Centre for Classification in Health. *The International Statistical Classification of Diseases and Related Health Problems*, 10th ed.; Australian modification (ICD-10-AM); National Centre for Classification in Health: Sydney, Australia, 1998.
30. Australian Bureau of Statistics, Australian Standard Geographical Classification (ASGC). *Statistical Geography*; Australian Bureau of Statistics: Canberra, Australia, 2006; Volume 1.
31. Australian Bureau of Statistics. *2033.0.55.001—Census of Population and Housing: Socio-Economic Indexes for Areas (SEIFA), Australia, 2011*; Australian Bureau of Statistics: Canberra, Australia, 2013. Available online: http://www.abs.gov.au/ausstats/abs@.nsf/Lookup/2033.0.55.001main+features100042011 (accessed on 7 July 2020).
32. Australian Bureau of Statistics. *2033.0.55.001—Census of Population and Housing: Socio-Economic Indexes for Areas (SEIFA), Australia, 2016*; Australian Bureau of Statistics: Canberra, Australia, 2018. Available online: https://www.abs.gov.au/ausstats/abs@.nsf/Lookup/by%20Subject/2033.0.55.001~{}2016~{}Main%20Features~{}IRSAD~{}20 (accessed on 7 July 2020).
33. Australian Bureau of Statistics. *Socio-Economic Indexes for Areas*; Australian Bureau of Statistics: Canberra, Australia, 2018. Available online: https://www.abs.gov.au/websitedbs/censushome.nsf/home/seifa (accessed on 5 November 2020).
34. Australian Bureau of Statistics. *Population—Australia*; Australian Bureau of Statistics: Canberra, Australia, 2020.
35. Australian Bureau of Statistics. *2011 Census QuickStats*; Australian Bureau of Statistics: Canberra, Australia, 2013. Available online: http://www.censusdata.abs.gov.au/census_services/getproduct/census/2011/quickstat/0?opendocument&navpos=220 (accessed on 5 November 2020).
36. Australian Bureau of Statistics. *2016 Census QuickStats*; Australian Government; Australian Bureau of Statistics: Canberra, Australia, 2017.
37. MEDCALC. *Medcalc—Relative Risk Calculator*; 2017; Available online: https://www.medcalc.org/calc/relative_risk.php (accessed on 5 November 2020).
38. IBM Corporation. *IBM SPSS Statistics for Windows Version 25*; IBM Corp: Armonk, NY, USA, 2010.
39. Keppel, G. *Design and Analysis: A Researcher's Handbook*, 3rd ed.; Prentice Hall: Englewood Cliffs, NJ, USA, 1991.
40. Peiris, S.; Berecki-Gisolf, J.; Chen, B.K.; Fildes, B. Road Trauma in Regional and Remote Australia and New Zealand in Preparedness for ADAS Technologies and Autonomous Vehicles. *Sustainability* **2020**, *12*, 4347. [CrossRef]
41. Franklin, R.C.; King, J.C.; Riggs, M. A Systematic Review of Large Agriculture Vehicles Use and Crash Incidents on Public Roads. *J. Agromed.* **2020**, *25*, 14–27. [CrossRef]
42. McKenzie, F. Population Decline in Non-Metropolitan Australia: Impacts and Policy Implications. *Urban Policy Res.* **1994**, *12*, 253–263. [CrossRef]
43. Wundersitz, L.; Palamara, P.; Brameld, K.; Raftery, S.; Thompson, J.; Govorko, M.; Watts, M. *Regional and Remote Road Safety: A National View*; Austroads: Canberra, Australia, 2019.
44. McGrail, M.R.; Humphreys, J.S. The index of rural access: An innovative integrated approach for measuring primary care access. *BMC Health Serv. Res.* **2009**, *9*, 124. [CrossRef]
45. Phillips, A. *Rural, Regional, and Remote Health: Indicators of Health Status and Determinants of Health*; Australian Institute of Health and Welfare: Canberra, Australia, 2008.
46. Armstrong, B.K.; Ba, J.A.G.; Leeder, S.R.; Rubin, G.L.; Russell, L.M. Challenges in health and health care for Australia. *Med. J. Aust.* **2007**, *187*, 485–489. [CrossRef]
47. Rachele, J.N.; Kavanagh, A.M.; Badland, H.; Giles-Corti, B.; Washington, S.; Turrell, G. Associations between individual socioeconomic position, neighbourhood disadvantage and transport mode: Baseline results from the HABITAT multilevel study. *J. Epidemiol. Community Health* **2015**, *69*, 1217–1223. [CrossRef]
48. Johns, M.; Lennon, A.; Haworth, N. Child Car Restraints:Mandating Type and Seating Row According to Age with Positive Effect in Regional City in Queensland, Australia. *Transp. Res. Rec.* **2012**, *2281*, 51–58. [CrossRef]

49. Rachele, J.N.; Learnihan, V.; Badland, H.M.; Mavoa, S.; Turrell, G.; Giles-Corti, B. Neighbourhood socioeconomic and transport disadvantage: The potential to reduce social inequities in health through transport. *J. Transp. Health* **2017**, *7*, 256–263. [CrossRef]
50. Wiesel, I.; Liu, F.; Buckle, C. Locational disadvantage and the spatial distribution of government expenditure on urban infrastructure and services in metropolitan Sydney (1988–2015). *Geogr. Res.* **2018**, *56*, 285–297. [CrossRef]
51. Rutter, P.A.; Behrendt, A.E. Adolescent suicide risk: Four psychosocial factors. *Adolescence* **2004**, *39*, 295. [PubMed]
52. Brent, D.A.; Baugher, M.; Bridge, J.; Chen, T.; Chiappetta, L. Age- and Sex-Related Risk Factors for Adolescent Suicide. *J. Am. Acad. Child Adolesc. Psychiatry* **1999**, *38*, 1497–1505. [CrossRef]
53. Zalsman, G.; Hawton, K.; Wasserman, D.; van Heeringen, K.; Arensman, E.; Sarchiapone, M.; Carli, V.; Höschl, C.; Barzilay, R.; Balazs, J.; et al. Suicide prevention strategies revisited: 10-year systematic review. *Lancet Psychiatry* **2016**, *3*, 646–659. [CrossRef]
54. Snowdon, J.; Harris, L. Firearms suicides in Australia. *Med. J. Aust.* **1990**, *156*, 79–83. [CrossRef]
55. Dudley, M.; Kelk, N.; Florio, T.; Waters, B.; Howard, J.; Taylor, D. Coroners' Records of Rural and Non-Rural Cases of Youth Suicide in New South Wales. *Aust. N. Z. J. Psychiatry* **1998**, *32*, 242–251. [CrossRef]
56. Cairns, J.-M.; Graham, E.; Bambra, C. Area-level socioeconomic disadvantage and suicidal behaviour in Europe: A systematic review. *Soc. Sci. Med.* **2017**, *192*, 102–111. [CrossRef]
57. Law, B.M.F.; Shek, D.T.L. A 6-year Longitudinal Study of Self-harm and Suicidal Behaviors among Chinese Adolescents in Hong Kong. *J. Pediatric Adolesc. Gynecol.* **2016**, *29* (Suppl. 1), S38–S48. [CrossRef]
58. Taylor, R.; Page, A.; Morrell, S.; Carter, G.; Harrison, J.E.; Carter, G. Socio-economic differentials in mental disorders and suicide attempts in Australia. *Br. J Psychiatry* **2004**, *185*, 486–493. [CrossRef]
59. Taylor, D.; Peden, A.E.; Franklin, R.C. Next steps for drowning prevention in rural and remote Australia: A systematic review of the literature. *Aust. J. Rural Health*. Available online: https://onlinelibrary.wiley.com/doi/abs/10.1111/ajr.12674 (accessed on 20 November 2020). [CrossRef]
60. Peden, A.E.; Willcox-Pidgeon, S.M.; Scarr, J.P.; Franklin, R.C. Comparing rivers to lakes: Implications for drowning prevention. *Aust. J. Rural Health*. Available online: https://onlinelibrary.wiley.com/doi/abs/10.1111/ajr.12679 (accessed on 24 November 2020). [CrossRef]
61. Peden, A.E.; Franklin, R.C.; Pearn, J.H. The prevention of child drowning: The causal factors and social determinants impacting fatalities in portable pools. *Health Promot. J. Aust.* **2020**, *31*, 184–191. [CrossRef] [PubMed]
62. Peden, A.E.; Barnsley, P.D.; Queiroga, A.C. The association between school holidays and unintentional fatal drowning among children and adolescents aged 5–17 years. *J. Paediatr. Child Health* **2018**, *55*, 533–538. [CrossRef] [PubMed]
63. Willcox-Pidgeon, S.M.; Peden, A.E.; Scarr, J. Exploring children's participation in commercial swimming lessons through the social determinants of health. *Health Promot. J. Aust.* **2020**, 1–10. [CrossRef] [PubMed]
64. Peden, A.E.; Franklin, R.C.; Leggat, P.A. Breathalysing and surveying river users in Australia to understand alcohol consumption and attitudes toward drowning risk. *BMC Public Health* **2018**, *18*, 1393. [CrossRef]
65. Ingram, G.; Kessides, C. Infrastructure for development. *J. Financ. Dev.* **1994**, *31*, 18.
66. Winschiers-Theophilus, H.; Winschiers-Goagoses, N.; Kasper Rodil, E.B.; Zaman, T.; Gereon Koch Kapuire, R.K. Moving away from Erindi-roukambe: Transferability of a rural community-based co-design. In Proceedings of the 12th International Conference on Social Implications of Computers in Developing Countries, Montego Bay, Jamaica, 19–22 May 2013.
67. Pawson, H.; Hulse, K.; Cheshire, L. *Addressing Concentrations of Disadvantage in Urban Australia*; Australian Housing and Urban Research Institute: Melbourne, Australia, 2015.
68. Peden, A.E.; Franklin, R.C.; Leggat, P.A. Cardiopulmonary resuscitation and first-aid training of river users in Australia: A strategy for reducing drowning. *Health Promot. J. Aust.* **2019**, *30*, 258–262. [CrossRef]
69. Cameron, P.; Dziukas, L.; Hadj, A.; Clark, P.; Hooper, S. Major Trauma in Australia: A Regional Analysis. *J. Trauma Acute Care Surg.* **1995**, *39*, 545–552. [CrossRef]

70. Fatovich, D.M.; Jacobs, I.G. The Relationship between Remoteness and Trauma Deaths in Western Australia. *J. Trauma* **2009**, *67*, 910–914. [CrossRef]
71. Australian Government Department of Health. *National Injury Prevention Strategy 2020–2030 (Draft for Consultation)*; Australian Government Department of Health: Canberra, Australia, 2020.

Publisher's Note: MDPI stays neutral with regard to jurisdictional claims in published maps and institutional affiliations.

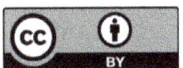

© 2020 by the authors. Licensee MDPI, Basel, Switzerland. This article is an open access article distributed under the terms and conditions of the Creative Commons Attribution (CC BY) license (http://creativecommons.org/licenses/by/4.0/).

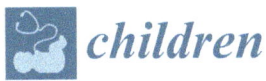

Article

Parent Mobile Phone Use in Playgrounds: A Paradox of Convenience

Keira Bury [1], Jonine Jancey [2] and Justine E. Leavy [2,*]

[1] School of Public Health, Curtin University, Perth 6845, WA, Australia; keira.bury@curtin.edu.au
[2] Collaboration for Evidence, Research and Impact in Public Health, School of Public Health, Faculty of Health Sciences, Curtin University, Perth 6845, WA, Australia; j.jancey@curtin.edu.au
* Correspondence: j.leavy@curtin.edu.au; Tel.: +61-8-9266-9285

Received: 17 October 2020; Accepted: 5 December 2020; Published: 10 December 2020

Abstract: Creating social and physical environments that promote good health is a key component of a social determinants approach. For the parents of young children, a smartphone offers opportunities for social networking, photography and multi-tasking. Understanding the relationship between supervision, mobile phone use and injury in the playground setting is essential. This research explored parent mobile device use (MDU), parent–child interaction in the playground, parent attitudes and perceptions towards MDU and strategies used to limit MDU in the playground. A mixed-methods approach collected naturalistic observations of parents of children aged 0–5 (n = 85) and intercept interviews (n = 20) at four metropolitan playgrounds in Perth, Western Australia. Most frequently observed MDU was scrolling (75.5%) and telephone calls (13.9%). Increased duration of MDU resulted in a reduction in supervision, parent–child play and increased child injury potential. The camera function offered the most benefits. Strategies to prevent MDU included turning to silent mode, wearing a watch and environmental cues. MDU was found to contribute to reduced supervision of children, which is a risk factor for injury. This is an emerging area of injury prevention indicating a need for broader strategies addressing the complex interplay between the social determinants and the developmental younger years.

Keywords: social determinants; children; child-play; mobile phone; injury; supervision

1. Introduction

For the parents of young children, a mobile device, such as a smartphone, offers opportunities for communication, social networking, photography, personal organisation, work flexibility and multi-tasking [1–4]. However, it can also be a source of distraction that brings about feelings of guilt and concern for poor role modelling of mobile device use (MDU) for young children during their early development [1,4–8]. Parent MDU can have detrimental effects on family relationships including interaction and attachment [3,5,9,10], reducing parents' responsiveness when children try to attract their attention [3,5] and social support [11].

The early years of life represent a vital time during which lifelong trajectories for health are determined by the complex interplay between the social determinants [12]. Social determinants of health are conditions in the environments in which children are born, live, learn, interact and play [13]. Creating social and physical environments that promote good health is a key component of a social determinants approach to health [14]. The social environment includes interactions with family and parent–child play encompasses social relationships in physical settings such as playgrounds [12,14,15]. Of interest, outdoor play is deemed fundamental for the physical, cognitive, emotional and social well-being of children [15,16], and has been declared a right of every child by the United Nations Convention on the Rights of the Child [17]. Outdoor play in early childhood has been linked to the social determinants that shape health and development, emphasising children's participation in play is influenced by multiple interacting social and contextual factors [15]. Very few studies have focused on understanding the social (e.g., parental supervision) and contextual (e.g., playground setting) factors that may influence behaviours and the relationship with the injury.

Whilst parent supervision is recognised as being a protective factor for injury in young children [18–20], there is evidence that there is a reduction in supervision quality as a result of parent MDU [21,22], and an association between parent MDU and injury in young children [23]. A recent US study found that children's safety needs were more often at risk when parents used their phones than when they were distracted by other factors, such as talking with other adults or reading printed material [24]. A review of the impact of parent MDU on parent–child interaction found increased phone ownership and related increases in parents' lack of attention to children could be associated with increases in childhood injuries [25]. US research has also reported a positive association between young children presenting at hospitals with injuries and the rapid adoption of smartphone use [23,26]. One study concluded that distraction from increased mobile phone use was directly associated with an increase in emergency hospitalisation for injuries in children aged 0–5 years; however, there was no association with children aged 6–10 years [23]. Hiniker et al. (2015), on the other hand, reported parents did not use their phone in the playground setting because they believed it would compromise their child's safety and lower their ability to respond. There is an increasing interest in understanding the impact of mobile device use by parents/carers of children aged 0–5 years [1,25], which commands an investigation into which characteristics of MDU are most absorbing of their attention [9,25,27] when supervising children.

The aim of the naturalistic study was twofold: first, to observe mode and duration of parent and caregiver MDU (telephone call, scroll/type or camera), parent/caregiver interaction and the coinciding behaviour (specifically: supervision, interaction and child injury) in the playground setting. Second, to explore parent/caregiver attitudes and perceptions of MDU and strategies used to limit MDU in the playground setting.

2. Materials and Methods

2.1. Study Design

A mixed-methods approach was used to collect quantitative and qualitative data from parent or caregiver/child dyads in playgrounds in Perth, Western Australia (WA). Trained researchers worked in teams of two to conduct covert, naturalistic observations ($n = 85$). In addition, intercept interviews were conducted with parents/caregivers ($n = 20$). The sample size for the observations was informed by naturalistic observational methodologies for data collection conducted in New South Wales, Australia ($n = 50$) [4] and New Jersey, US ($n = 60$) [27], whilst one other study in the US collected 171 observations over almost double (seven parks) [24] compared with four in this study. The sample size for the interview numbers ($n = 20$) were consistent with similar studies [4,27].

2.2. Study Setting

The study was undertaken in four playgrounds across a range of Socio-Economic Indexes for Areas (SEIFA) [28] in metropolitan Perth, WA. The playgrounds included: (i) a fenced playground with several different play areas, built specifically for 6-year-olds and under; (ii) a fenced playground with low-level equipment for toddlers; (iii) an ungated single playground adjacent to a number of BBQ pits, and grass/benches for picnics; and (iv) an ungated single playground. Observations were undertaken on school days between the hours of 9:30 a.m. and 12:30 p.m., a time when older siblings have been dropped off at school and a popular time for 0–5 years to attend playgrounds [4,27].

2.3. Study Participants

Participants were parent or caregiver/child dyads where the parent/caregiver appeared to be under 45 years, attending the playground by themselves (not with another adult) and caring for at least one independently mobile child who appeared to be under 5 years. The estimation of the child's age was based on general appearance and height. Parents caring for more than one child were included in the study. Where parent/carers had multiple children under their care, the researchers chose the child that best fitted the criteria—under 5 years and independently mobile. Participants were not notified they were being observed so as to obtain naturalistic data. Participants who left the playground or were lost from the site (into a café/toilet) within the first 10 min of the observation were excluded from the study. Researchers recruited participants for intercept interviews ($n = 20$). Parent/Carers appearing to meet the participant criteria were approached and invited to participate in the study. No parent/carers declined to be interviewed. Participants were provided with an information sheet and consent form prior to the commencement of interviews. Ethics approval was obtained for this study by Curtin University Research Ethics Committee no: HRE2016-0027.

2.4. Quantitative and Qualitative Data Collection

2.4.1. Quantitative

The two researchers positioned themselves within the boundary of the playground to observe participants, one observation at a time. At the beginning of the observation period, the researchers synchronised stopwatches to concurrently record data for a period of up to twenty minutes. Participants were observed for MDU (mode and duration of use), caregiver supervision, caregiver/child interaction and child injury potential with data recorded during each minute.

The first researcher collected data for caregiver MDU using an adapted, previously trialled mobile device timing audit [4,27]. During each minute of the observation, the researcher observed the dominant mode of caregiver MDU (telephone call, scroll/type or camera) and the duration of caregiver MDU (recorded as a minimum of 0 s and a maximum of 60 s). The summed duration for each minute of observation was later categorised as; "No MDU"; "1–10 s"; "11–20 s"; "21–30 s"; "31–40 s"; "41–50 s" and "51–60 s". The second researcher collected data on caregiver supervision, caregiver–child interaction and child injury potential using a combined observation audit [4,27]. During each minute of the observation, the researcher observed and recorded the dominant behaviour.

2.4.2. Qualitative

Caregivers appearing to meet the participant criteria were approached and invited to participate in the study. Participants were provided with an information sheet and consent form prior to the commencement of interviews. The researcher recorded the intercept interviews using a structured interview schedule. Each interview took approximately 10 min to complete. The interviews were conducted by two researchers, field notes were kept by both researchers and compared for consistency at the completion of each interview period.

2.5. Measures

Data from the mobile timing device audit were collapsed and used to create three categorical variables:

(1) MDU: this binary variable categorised minutes as either "No MDU" (0 s of MDU) or "MDU" (1–60 s of MDU).
(2) MDU Mode: this variable categorised minutes as "Telephone call" (using the device telephone call function) "Scroll/type" (using the device touchscreen function), or "Camera" (using the device camera function).
(3) MDU Duration: this variable categorised the summed MDU duration for each minute as "No MDU" (0 s of observed), "1–10 s", "11–20 s", "21–30 s", "31–40 s", "41–50 s", "51–60 s" (of observed MDU).

Data from the caregiver–child observation tool for supervision, interaction and injury potential were collapsed:

(1) Supervision: "Constant supervision" (caregiver watching, following, mediating, redirecting the child or remaining in close proximity); "Intermittent supervision" (caregiver sought visual contact with the child intermittently); "No supervision" (caregiver had no contact with the child).
(2) Interaction: "Caregiver-child play" (caregiver and child play together), "Independent play" (child plays without caregiver), "Verbal interaction" (caregiver and/or child talking or calling to each other), "Hold/touch" (physical contact between caregiver and child), "Sitting/eating/drinking" (caregiver and child in close proximity having a drink or food).
(3) Injury Potential: Child injury risk was measured using an adapted injury risk behaviour checklist developed by Dotson (2013). Injury potential was categorised as "Increased injury" potential (unsafe play behaviours, i.e., child passes within moving radius of equipment, child uses equipment in an unintended manner), "Decreased injury" potential (safe play behaviours, i.e., child takes precaution, child stops swing and dismounts) or "Inadequate carer supervision" (i.e., child moves out of view of caregiver, the caregiver does not give child direction on how to behave safely).

2.6. Analysis

2.6.1. Quantitative Data

The data for the 85 observed participants were broken down into one-minute blocks which resulted in a total of 1532 min of observation time which was entered into SPSS version 23 [29]. Descriptive statistics were used to describe the parent/caregiver participant characteristics and the children under the parent/caregiver's supervision. The quantitative analysis explored the coinciding MDU, supervision, interaction and injury risk behaviours within each minute of the observation. A series of cross-tabulations with Pearson chi-square tests with a significance level of $p < 0.01$ were conducted to test the association between MDU, MDU Mode, MDU Duration and the outcome variables Supervision, Interaction and Injury Potential.

2.6.2. Qualitative Data Collection and Analysis

The interviews were transcribed verbatim by one researcher (KB) and were divided among the research team for open coding (KB, JL, JJ). The first researcher then collated the coded interviews using NVIVO 12 [30] and identified relationships between the codes to form the emerging themes which were agreed upon by the research team. Data saturation was reached during the data collection process ($n = 20$) and no new concepts emerged. Identified themes were consistent with work previously undertaken by Australian researchers [4]. The general inductive approach is a straightforward easily used, systematic set of procedures for analysing qualitative data and provides reliable findings [31]. Participant quotes to support the themes have been de-identified and presented in the results.

3. Results

3.1. Playground Observations

3.1.1. Participant Characteristics

Participants were mostly female ($n = 72$, 85%) and caring for one child under the age of 5 years ($n = 68$, 80%). Of the 85 parent/caregiver–child dyad observations ($n = 85$), 47 were in high socio-economic status (SES) playground locations and 38 in low SES playground locations.

3.1.2. Mobile Device Use—Mode and Duration

During the observation period, caregiver MDU was observed among 70% ($n = 59$) of the caregiver–child dyads, 30% ($n = 16$) of parents/carers did not use their mobile device, with total caregiver MDU comprising 23.5% of the observed time. The most frequently observed mode of MDU was "Scrolling/typing" ($n = 272$, 75.5%), followed by telephone call ($n = 50$, 13.9%) and using the camera ($n = 38$, 10.5%). The duration of MDU was either short of "1–10 s" ($n = 91$) or almost a full minute ("51–60 s") ($n = 92$).

3.1.3. Caregiver Mobile Device Use and Caregiver Supervision

Table 1 presents a comparison of supervision behaviours between minutes of "No MDU" and minutes of "MDU". For all observed minutes, the proportion of "No supervision" was higher when using a mobile device (MDU) compared with "No MDU" (29.4% and 5.2%, respectively). The proportion of "Constant supervision" was similar for "MDU" (45.8%) and "No MDU" (43.6%). A significant association was found between MDU and caregiver supervision $\chi^2(2) = 191.67, p \leq 0.001$.

Table 1. Caregiver supervision by minutes of no mobile device use (No MDU) compared with minutes of mobile device use (MDU).

Caregiver Supervision *	No MDU		MDU		Total	
	n	%	n	%	n	%
Constant supervision	511	43.6	165	45.8	676	44.1
Intermittent supervision	600	51.2	89	24.7	689	45.0
No supervision	61	5.2	106	29.4	167	10.9

* $p \leq 0.001$.

3.1.4. Caregiver Mobile Device Use and Caregiver–Child Interaction

"Independent play" (32.6%, $n = 500$) and "Caregiver–child play" (35.4%, $n = 542$) each made up one-third of the interaction behaviour of all observed minutes (Table 2). However, the proportion of "Caregiver–child play" with MDU was half that of no MDU (20.3% and 40.0%, respectively), while the proportion of "Independent play" for MDU was double that of "No MDU" (50.3% compared with 27.2%, respectively). The results show similar proportions for "Verbal interaction" within the "MDU" and "No MDU" groups (22.2% and 20.8%, respectively). A significant association was found between MDU and caregiver–child interaction $\chi^2(4) = 81.95, p \leq 0.001$.

Table 2. Caregiver–child interaction by minutes of no mobile device use (No MDU) compared with minutes of mobile device use (MDU).

Caregiver–Child Interaction *	No MDU		MDU		Total	
	n	%	n	%	n	%
Caregiver–child play	469	40.0	73	20.3	542	35.4
Verbal interaction	244	20.8	80	22.2	324	21.1
Hold/touch	75	6.4	11	3.1	86	5.6
Sitting/eating/drinking	65	5.5	15	4.2	80	5.2
Independent play	319	27.2	181	50.3	500	32.6

* $p \leq 0.001$.

3.1.5. Caregiver Mobile Device Use and Child Injury Potential

Increased child injury potential was observed among 9.5% ($n = 146$) of all observed minutes. The proportion of observed "Increased injury potential" for "No MDU" was 5.7% ($n = 67$) compared with 21.9% ($n = 79$) with "MDU" (Table 3). The highest proportion of "Increased injury potential" was observed in the "51–60 s" ($n = 30$, 32.6%) MDU duration category. When comparing child injury potential across the mode of caregiver MDU, the highest proportion of "Increased injury potential" was observed for "Telephone call" ($n = 13$, 26%).

Table 3. Child injury potential by minutes of no mobile device use (No MDU) compared with minutes of mobile device use (MDU).

Child Injury Potential	No MDU		MDU		Total	
	n	%	n	%	n	%
Decreased	1105	94.3	281	78.1	1386	90.5
Increased	67	5.7	79	21.9	146	9.5
	1172	100.0	360	100.0	1532	100.0

3.2. Playground Interviews

3.2.1. Participant Characteristics

Interviewed participants (Table 4) were mostly female ($n = 15$, 75%), born in Australia ($n = 12$, 60%), university educated ($n = 14$, 70%) and supervising one child ($n = 14$, 70%) with a mean age of 2.5 years.

Table 4. Demographic characteristics of interview participants ($n = 20$).

Characteristic	n	%
Sex		
Female	15	75
Male	5	25
Age (years)		
25–29	4	20
30–34	9	45
35–39	3	15
40+	4	20
Country of birth		
Australia	12	60
Other	8	40
Highest level of education		
Year 12 or Equivalent	1	5
Trade/Diploma	5	25
Bachelor Degree or higher	14	70
Working status		
In paid work	10	50
Not in paid work	10	50

3.2.2. Reported MDU Behaviours

Almost all participants reported using their mobile device at the playground that day ($n = 19$, 95%). Participants made short statements around their reason for their MDU in the playground on that day such as *"Had to answer a couple of business calls"* (P13) and *"Just to check if I've received any messages"* (P21). The most frequently reported reason for MDU included methods of communications (calls, text, email) ($n = 12$, 60%). Other reasons included photography ($n = 9$, 45%) and using the device to undertake specific tasks for personal administration ($n = 3$, 15%).

3.2.3. Perspectives on Caregiver MDU

Four dominant themes emerged from the participant interviews; these were: convenience, distraction, security and making memories.

3.2.4. Convenience

Participants cited essential daily communication including telephone calls and text-messaging, connecting through social media networks, easy access to information, and photography, for example,

"If you need to know where a street is you can just google it. Taking photos of my child, sending them to different people would be an advantage and most importantly, if there's an emergency I can call someone." (P19).

In addition, other activities were web browsing for news, sports scores, attending to work-related matters, or activities for personal "admin", such as banking, shopping and coordinating services such as car repairs. The ability to undertake these activities anytime, anywhere *"I guess you can multitask, you can get those little things done when you have a chance"* (P20) contributed to the convenience and the need to carry a mobile device.

3.2.5. Distraction

In contrast, most participants reported that notifications, social media and the obligation to check in with work were a distraction, for example, *"If you've got your phone it's very easy to be distracted and to keep it constantly in use and to be distracted from doing this I'll just check Facebook."* (P2) Whilst the obligation to check in with work was also a distraction, *"You can feel obligated to check work emails, like I'm just stepping out of work for today just to watch him for a minute but you do feel obligated to be checking, too available."* (P5).

Participants highlighted a paradox between the convenience and distraction of MDU, giving reasons why they would not use their device in the playground. For example:

"I guess that you have to be conscious that it doesn't distract you from spending this time with the kids ..., and giving them your full attention because you want to be interacting, you want to be there with them in the moment". (P20) However, there was a tension between distraction and convenience, *"It's like a psychological kind of thing where I'm drawn to answer that beep and that takes me away from my kid. It's on silent now. It's just a distraction. I use it for my convenience rather than other people's convenience."* (P16).

Participants believed that brief moments of MDU, such as making a telephone call would have the least impact on supervision, whereas lengthy periods viewing the device for text messaging or social media were more likely to diminish the quality of supervision, *"I think if you're scrolling through Facebook, then that obviously requires a lot more attention than if you're communicating on a phone. I think you're much more able to supervise if you're only using it in its basic sense whereas if you're typing a text or you're writing an email, scrolling through Facebook then I think your ability to supervise is impaired. Coz obviously it takes more concentration."* (P5).

Using the camera was viewed differently *"Other than photos, anytime you are with your kids you should be supervising them so in public unless you've got somebody else with you who can take over that role. I always have eyes on (child) even through the camera on my phone. I think that's the main thing."* (P16).

Participants commented on the social acceptability of MDU within the playground setting with work tasks or essential telephone calls deemed more acceptable distractions than social media, along with some criticism of this behaviour. For example, *"There's not too many things that are more important than watching a kid, you know if he's close to the road you don't need to use your phone but if he's in the playground and I need to take a phone call for any particular reason. But I don't think there is any reason that you need to use Facebook or something like that if the kid needs watching."* (P5).

3.2.6. Security

Participants frequently reported the benefit ($n = 14$, 70%) of having their mobile device in case of an emergency within the playground, *"The phone is just there as a secondary device as an emergency or if you need to contact someone."* (P21); or outside the playground setting, *"I really just try not to answer your phone unless you absolutely have to. You don't want to miss a call either, if it's something important like family or an emergency."* (P18).

When considering supervising children, participants made comparisons to other settings, for example, being in and around water, *"She actually just turned around to talk to me for a few seconds and that's all it took for a one year old to nose dive into the pool ... I think so much can happen in the blink of an eyelid, you can't take your eye off them."* (P18). Or other settings like driving a car, *"You can't *have your eyes on two things at once, it's impossible. Other people maybe can, I don't think I can. It's like the driving, they wouldn't have it banned if it were safe. Surely."* (P22).

3.2.7. Making Memories

Photography was highlighted as a valuable aspect of MDU which enhanced their experience at the playground, *"To capture precious moments, to be in contact with other people that aren't with you. Family overseas, you can post a photo of Facebook they can kind of be a part of it as well."* (P10) It enabled them to capture memories with their children and share these with loved ones at a later date.

Caregivers were concerned about the ability to interact with and supervise children while using a mobile device, particularly if it involved using social media. However, photography was commonly indicated as an acceptable mode of MDU in the playground indicating the perception that photography can both mitigate safety concerns and enable interaction with children. For example: *"I'm supposed to be looking after her, engaging with her, supervising her and making sure that she's safe unless it's for the camera."* (P16).

3.2.8. Strategies for Limiting MDU around Children

Caregivers were forthcoming about their desire to limit MDU, which stemmed from wanting to spend quality time with their child, avoid distraction in risky settings, and role model appropriate technology use, so as to not raise device focussed children.

All participants nominated strategies to limit their MDU use in the playground setting, with the most common strategy defined as abstinence, *"Don't bring it out, don't bring it, wear a watch!"* (P6). Other participants, however, referred to restricting the functionality of their device by putting it on silence or only using it for a camera, *"Put it on silent. I don't have my phone on when I'm meant to be watching her because I know how quickly things can change as well. Also having it on silent I don't kind of have that niggling feeling to look at all the beeps that go off. Just think of it as a camera when you're at the park, nothing else."* (P16).

Participants reported 'downtime', which were times when they perceived their child was occupied and required less supervision or interaction. One participant explained *"Most things require you to look at the screen. When she's on the swing. I'm not as concerned, coz she's strapped in, she's holding on. I look at it frequently, don't get me wrong, I'm not some saint."* (P15).

Some participants reported the need to role-model positive MDU behaviours for their children, *"I don't really think they need to come out of your bag when you're at the playground or at schools or in social situations with your own friends, you should be engaging with the people there in front of you. Family mealtimes, it's really important to sit down together, have dinner, have a discussion. I think kids today will miss out on a lot of social skills if they see everyone on their smartphone all the time."* (P19). This resulted in curbing their MDU.

4. Discussion

This naturalistic study explored mobile device use by parent/caregivers of children aged 0–5 years in four playgrounds in metropolitan Perth, Western Australia. The study found that parent texting/scrolling, telephone calls and camera use were a common occurrence in the playground setting (70% of observation participants) but occupied a small part of their time at the playground. This finding is consistent with other research in Australia and the US [4,27], however, the paradox between convenience and distraction was a salient theme of the study which has also been found in other research [7,24,32,33]. Of interest, parents and carers suggested that the practicality of having a mobile phone close-by was reassuring in the event of an emergency, thus creating a tension between having the mobile phone close by or not at all. Child-injury prevention agencies and playground designers should explore broad strategies to promote the importance of supervision to prevent child injury, reduction in MDU in social settings and the promotion of parent–child play. Going forward, policies and programmes must embrace the social determinants of health that play a vital role in the development years.

It has been suggested that the longer the time spent on a mobile device, increases the negative impact on supervision, and decreases interaction with the child [24]. This finding was supported by our observations, for as the time on the mobile device increased, the supervision and caregiver–child play decreased, being replaced by no parent/carer supervision, and independent play by the child. Furthermore, when parents were on the mobile device for a full minute, the potential for injury increased, compared with those parent/carers not using their mobile device. The injury potential increased when the supervision was interrupted by scrolling and increased again when on a telephone call. There is recent evidence suggesting children's safety needs are compromised when parents use their mobile phones [34], and smartphone ownership by parents' may help explain the increase in young children presenting at ED with injuries [23,26]. Interviewees acknowledged the potential for interrupted supervision, especially if there was an opportunity to multi-task (e.g., telephone calls or check work emails). However, worthy of exploration is the notion that a parent/carer may take the child to the playground more frequently because they can use their smartphone to multi-task, e.g., access e-mails, and in turn the child may get injured more, not because the caregiver is distracted but simply because the child goes to the playground more [23]. Our findings support a recent review where parents reported the need for uninterrupted supervision of children in and around playgrounds, roads and waterways where there is the potential for childhood injury [25]. Further research to fully understand the level of device distraction, multi-tasking and childhood safety to provide guidelines for parents' use is a research priority.

This study found that the tasks (telephone call, scroll/type or camera) undertaken on the mobile device influenced supervision and the opportunity for the social interplay between parents and their children. Participants reported that scrolling/texting resulted in a break from visual supervision, however, using the camera function not only maintained supervision but was often associated with play interaction between parents and their child. Of interest, parent/caregivers did not connect camera use with being distracted, and this finding is consistent with another recent Australian study that found parents value mobile devices as a way to capture memorable moments [4]. Noteworthy, the longer the time spent on taking or making a telephone call was found to be most closely associated with no supervision and minimal play between the parent and the child. Parental behaviours have a critical role as a social determinant of child development. For example, positive reinforcement while on play equipment, displays of warmth and affection result in fewer child behaviour problems and positive peer relations that, in turn, enhance a child's health [12]. An investment in early child development as a determinant of health will translate to learning skills and increased well-being across the life course.

Using a social determinants lens, early childhood development opportunities are affected by various social and environmental factors, including relationships with parents and caregivers [12]. The playground, specifically controlled, gated playground environments purpose-built for those under 6 years of age, provide co-benefits for the child and parent/carer. There is an opportunity for children's involvement in independent, active and risky play [34–36]; and a time for parents to 'take a break' from constant supervision acknowledging that some minor injuries are an inevitable aspect of early childhood [37]. As such, factors including a child's age, physical ability and the playground design have the potential to influence the level and type of supervision, and the benefit of parents using their mobile device whilst at the playground. Furthermore, recent literature supporting risky play, i.e., a play that is thrilling and exciting but includes the possibility of physical injury, has been positively associated with physical and social health in children [36]. However, despite the differing designs of the four playgrounds in this study, ranging from a large gated setting with multiple play areas to a small single ungated play area, similar patterns of MDU and supervision were observed. Further exploration of the mitigation of potential risks of MDU and the interplay of the benefits might be an area worthy of future research.

Social acceptability and parent role-modelling were identified as influences of parent MDU. Quick calls, text messages and work were deemed more acceptable than using the device for social media or entertainment. Observations of other adults MDU in the playground were reported to influence interviewee's attitudes to their own MDU and how this relates to 'good parenting' but also the importance of role-modelling non-intentional use [27] to their children and to other adults in the playground setting. These perspectives contrast to prior work where caregivers were less critical of others and reserved judgement about the appropriateness of others' MDU [27]. These findings may highlight a changing social climate that is becoming more critical of parent/caregiver MDU and may indicate a need for realistic population-wide strategies to raise awareness of the risks associated with the distraction caused by mobile phones.

Most interviewees indicated that they had experienced success in limiting their own MDU and offered a range of strategies to help minimise use when caring for children. These strategies included abstinence, achieved by leaving the device in a bag, at home or in the car, choosing a phone function mode such as a silent or camera, and synchronising MDU during times when they perceived children required less interaction or supervision. In addition, a less often mentioned but observed strategy was caregiver proximal supervision i.e., following the child around the playground and keeping close whilst using a mobile device. This behaviour enabled the caregiver to maintain 'Constant supervision' whilst engaging in MDU [20]; however, it did not support caregiver–child interaction and exploit the time for parents and children to interact in a play setting.

Strengths and Limitations

To our knowledge, this is the first research to examine an association between the characteristics of parent/caregiver MDU (duration and mode) and caregiver–child interaction, caregiver supervision and child injury potential, providing new evidence. A mixed-method approach provided a range of perspectives and strategies that parents use to limit their MDU around children. There were a number of limitations including: an over-representation of females; small sample size, however, this is consistent with other similar research [4,24,27]. The approximate age of the child in the parent/child dyad was not estimated (other than being under 5 years), so we did not have an approximated age break down to complete any additional analysis by age, and half of the playgrounds being located in higher SES, metropolitan areas.

5. Conclusions

The majority of caregivers reported that whilst MDU was convenient for communication, personal organisation and security, it was an unwanted distraction in the playground, where supervising and interacting with children should be the priority. However, the exception was the camera, which was highly valued by caregivers for making memories and also offered the most support for maintaining supervision and interaction through play. Mobile device use was found to contribute to reduced supervision of children, which is a risk factor for injury. This is an emerging area of injury prevention that indicates the need for broader strategies addressing the complex interplay that exists between the social determinants and the developmental younger years. Finally, the caregiver perspectives from this research are valuable for the development of realistic and effective strategies that support parents and caregivers to achieve their desired MDU.

Author Contributions: J.J. and J.E.L. conceived the research design and K.B. participated in design and coordination. K.B. collected, cleaned and analysed the data and drafted the manuscript. J.J. and J.E.L. were responsible for initial coding, critically revising the manuscript, editing and providing guidance on the manuscript. K.B., J.J. and J.E.L. read and approved the final paper. All authors have read and agreed to the published version of the manuscript.

Funding: This research received no external funding.

Acknowledgments: We would like to thank the participants of the study.

Conflicts of Interest: The authors declare no conflict of interest.

References

1. Hiniker, A. *Supporting Intentional Media Use in Families*; Kientz, J.A., Aragon, C., Munson, S., Eds.; ProQuest Dissertations Publishing: New York, NY, USA, 2017.
2. Ferguson, M.; Carlson, D.; Boswell, W.; Whitten, D.; Butts, M.M.; Kacmar, K.M.; Thompson, M.J. Tethered to work: A family systems approach linking mobile device use to turnover intentions. *J. Appl. Psychol.* **2016**, *101*, 520–534. [CrossRef]
3. Radesky, J.S.; Kistin, C.J.; Zuckerman, B.; Nitzberg, K.; Gross, J.; Kaplan-Sanoff, M.; Augustyn, M.; Silverstein, M. Patterns of mobile device use by caregivers and children during meals in fast food restaurants. *Pediatrics* **2014**, *133*, e843. [CrossRef]
4. Mangan, E.; Leavy, J.; Jancey, J.M. Mobile device use when caring for children 0-5 years: A naturalistic playground study. *Health Promot. J. Aust.* **2018**, *29*, 337–343. [CrossRef]
5. Blackman, A. *Screen Time for Parents and Caregivers: Parental Screen Distraction and Parenting Perceptions and Beliefs*; Mowder, B., Ed.; Pace University: New York, NY, USA, 2015.
6. Radesky, J.S.; Kistin, C.; Eisenberg, S.; Gross, J.; Block, G.; Zuckerman, B.; Silverstein, M. Parent Perspectives on Their Mobile Technology Use: The Excitement and Exhaustion of Parenting While Connected. *J. Dev. Behav. Pediatr.* **2016**, *37*, 694–701. [CrossRef]
7. McDaniel, B.T.; Coyne, S.M. Technology interference in the parenting of young children: Implications for mothers' perceptions of coparenting. *Soc. Sci. J.* **2016**, *53*, 435–443. [CrossRef]
8. Mehrotra, S.; Tripathi, R. Recent developments in the use of smartphone interventions for mental health. *Curr. Opin. Psychiatry* **2018**, *31*, 379–388. [CrossRef] [PubMed]
9. Ante-Contreras, D. *Distracted Parenting: How Social Media Affects Parent-Child Attachment*; California State University: San Bernardino, CA, USA, 2016; p. 292.
10. Carlson, D.S.; Thompson, M.J.; Crawford, W.S.; Boswell, W.R.; Whitten, D. Your job is messing with mine! The impact of mobile device use for work during family time on the spouse's work life. *J. Occup. Health Psychol.* **2018**, *23*, 471–482. [CrossRef] [PubMed]
11. Reimers, A.K.; Boxberger, K.; Schmidt, S.; Niessner, C.; Demetriou, Y.; Marzi, I.; Woll, A. Social Support and Modelling in Relation to Physical Activity Participation and Outdoor Play in Preschool Children. *Children* **2019**, *6*, 115. [CrossRef] [PubMed]
12. Maggi, S.; Irwin, L.J.; Siddiqi, A.; Hertzman, C. The social determinants of early child development: An overview. *J. Paediatr. Child Health* **2010**, *46*, 627–635. [CrossRef]
13. Marmot, M.; Friel, S.; Bell, R.; Houweling, T.A.J.; Taylor, S. Closing the gap in a generation: Health equity through action on the social determinants of health. *Lancet* **2008**, *372*, 1661–1669. [CrossRef]
14. Healthy People 2020: An Opportunity to Address the Societal Determinants of Health in the United States. Available online: http://www.healthypeople.gov/2010/hp2020/advisory/SocietalDeterminantsHealth.htm (accessed on 1 October 2020).
15. Parent, N.; Guhn, M.; Brussoni, M.; Almas, A.; Oberle, E. Social determinants of playing outdoors in the neighbourhood: Family characteristics, trust in neighbours and daily outdoor play in early childhood. *Can. J. Public Health* **2020**, 1–8. [CrossRef] [PubMed]
16. Ginsburg, K.R. The importance of play in promoting healthy child development and maintaining strong parent-child bonds. *Pediatrics* **2007**, *119*, 182–191. [CrossRef] [PubMed]
17. McGoldrick, D. The united nations convention on the rights of the child. *Int. J. Law Policy Fam.* **1991**, *5*, 132–169. [CrossRef]
18. Schnitzer, P.G.; Dowd, M.D.; Kruse, R.L.; Morrongiello, B.A. Supervision and risk of unintentional injury in young children. *Inj. Prev.* **2015**, *21*, e63–e70. [CrossRef] [PubMed]
19. Schwebel, D.C. Safety on the Playground: Mechanisms Through Which Adult Supervision Might Prevent Child Playground Injury. *J. Clin. Psychol. Med. Settings* **2006**, *13*, 135–143. [CrossRef]
20. Saluja, G.; Brenner, R.A.; Morrongiello, B.A.; Haynie, D.; Rivera, M.; Cheng, T.L. The role of supervision in child injury risk: Definition, conceptual and measurement issues. *Inj. Control Saf. Promot.* **2004**, *11*, 17–22. [CrossRef] [PubMed]
21. Moran, K. Watching Parents, Watching Kids: Water Safety Supervision of Young Children at the Beach. *Int. J. Aquat. Res. Educ.* **2010**, *4*, 269–277. [CrossRef]

22. Simon, H.K.; Tamura, T.; Colton, K. Reported level of supervision of young children while in the bathtub. *Ambul. Pediatr.* **2003**, *3*, 106–108. [CrossRef]
23. Palsson, C. Smartphones and child injuries. *J. Public Econ.* **2017**, *156*, 200–213. [CrossRef]
24. Lemish, D.; Elias, N.; Floegel, D. "Look at me!" Parental use of mobile phones at the playground. *Mob. Media Commun.* **2019**, *8*, 170–187. [CrossRef]
25. Kildare, C.A.; Middlemiss, W. Impact of parents mobile device use on parent-child interaction: A literature review. *Comput. Hum. Behav.* **2017**, *75*, 579–593. [CrossRef]
26. The Perils of Texting While Parenting. Available online: http://members.aon.at/emarsale/deutsch/Perils_of_texting.pdf (accessed on 28 May 2018).
27. Hiniker, A.; Sobel, K.; Suh, H. *Texting while Parenting: How Adults Use Mobile Phones while Caring for Children at the Playground*; Association for Computing Machinery: New York, NY, USA, 2015; pp. 727–736.
28. Australian Bureau of Statistics. *Census of Population and Housing: Socio-Economic Indexes for Areas (SEIFA) 2016*; ABS: Canberra, Australia, 2016.
29. IBM Corp. *IBM SPSS Statistics for Windows, version 23.0.*; IBM Corp: Arnmork, NY, USA, 2015.
30. NVivo Qualitative Data Analysis Software. Available online: https://www.qsrinternational.com/nvivo-qualitative-data-analysis-software/home (accessed on 28 May 2018).
31. Thomas, D.R. A General Inductive Approach for Analyzing Qualitative Evaluation Data. *Am. J. Eval.* **2006**, *27*, 237–246. [CrossRef]
32. Jarvenpaa, S.L.; Lang, K.R. Managing the Paradoxes of Mobile Technology. *Inf. Syst. Manag.* **2005**, *22*, 7–23. [CrossRef]
33. Oduor, E.; Neustaedter, C.; Odom, W.; Tang, A.; Moallem, N.; Tory, M.; Irani, P. The Frustrations and Benefits of Mobile Device Usage in the Home when Co-Present with Family Members. In Proceedings of the 2016 ACM Conference on Designing Interactive Systems, Brisbane, Australia, 4–6 June 2016; Association for Computing Machinery: New York, NY, USA, 2016; pp. 1315–1327.
34. Mitchell, R.J.; Cavanagh, M.; Eager, D. Not all risk is bad, playgrounds as a learning environment for children. *Int. J. Inj. Control. Saf. Promot.* **2006**, *13*, 122–124. [CrossRef] [PubMed]
35. Lee, H.; Tamminen, K.A.; Clark, A.M.; Slater, L.; Spence, J.C.; Holt, N. A meta-study of qualitative research examining determinants of children's independent active free play. *Int. J. Behav. Nutr. Phys. Act.* **2015**, *12*, 5. [CrossRef]
36. Brussoni, M.; Gibbons, R.; Gray, C.; Ishikawa, T.; Sandseter, E.B.H.; Bienenstock, A.; Chabot, G.; Fuselli, P.; Herrington, S.; Janssen, I.; et al. What is the Relationship between Risky Outdoor Play and Health in Children? A Systematic Review. *Int. J. Environ. Res. Public Health* **2015**, *12*, 6423–6454. [CrossRef]
37. Ablewhite, J.; Peel, I.; McDaid, L.; Hawkins, A.; Goodenough, T.; Deave, T.; Stewart, J.; Kendrick, D. Parental perceptions of barriers and facilitators to preventing child unintentional injuries within the home: A qualitative study. *BMC Public Health* **2015**, *15*, 280. [CrossRef]

Publisher's Note: MDPI stays neutral with regard to jurisdictional claims in published maps and institutional affiliations.

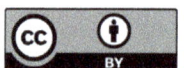

© 2020 by the authors. Licensee MDPI, Basel, Switzerland. This article is an open access article distributed under the terms and conditions of the Creative Commons Attribution (CC BY) license (http://creativecommons.org/licenses/by/4.0/).

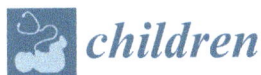

Article

Work-Related Fatalities Involving Children in New Zealand, 1999–2014

Rebbecca Lilley [1,*], Bronwen McNoe [1], Gabrielle Davie [1], Brandon de Graaf [1] and Tim Driscoll [2]

[1] Injury Prevention Research Unit, Otago Medical School, University of Otago, 9054 Dunedin, New Zealand; bronwen.mcnoe@otago.ac.nz (B.M.); gabrielle.davie@otago.ac.nz (G.D.); brandon.degraaf@otago.ac.nz (B.d.G.)
[2] School of Public Health, Faculty of Medicine and Health, The University of Sydney, Sydney, NSW 2006, Australia; tim.driscoll@sydney.edu.au
* Correspondence: rebbecca.lilley@otago.ac.nz; Tel.: +64-3479-7230

Received: 30 November 2020; Accepted: 22 December 2020; Published: 24 December 2020

Abstract: In high income countries, children under 15 years of age are exposed to workplace hazards when they visit or live on worksites or participate in formal or informal work. This study describes the causes and circumstances of unintentional child work-related fatal injuries (child WRFI) in New Zealand. Potential cases were identified from the Mortality Collection using International Classification of Disease external cause codes: these were matched to Coronial records and reviewed for work-relatedness. Data were abstracted on the socio-demographic, employment and injury-related circumstances. Of the 1335 unintentional injury deaths in children from 1999 through 2014, 206 (15%) were identified as dying from a work-related injury: 9 workers and 197 bystanders—the majority involving vehicle crashes or being stuck by moving objects in incidents occurring on farms or public roads. Those at highest risk were males, preschoolers, and those of Māori or European ethnicity. Work made a notable contribution to the burden of unintentional fatal injury in children with most deaths highly preventable, largely by adult intervention and legislation. To address the determinants of child WRFI greater attention on rural farm and transport settings would result in a significant reduction in the injury mortality rates of New Zealand children.

Keywords: injury; work; children; agriculture; farm; transport; occupational injury

1. Introduction

Unintentional injury is a leading cause of premature mortality in New Zealand children aged 1–14 years, accounting for two in five deaths in this age group [1–3]. Child injury mortality is inequitably distributed in New Zealand [3]. There are clear disparities for New Zealand's indigenous Māori children who experience a rate of fatal injury 3.5 times greater than that for non-Māori children [1]. New Zealand's child injury mortality rate is amongst the poorest amongst comparative Organisation for Economic Co-operation and Development (OECD) nations, being more than twice the rate of Sweden, the United Kingdom, Netherlands and Italy [4]. A 2009 report card scoring the adoption and implementation of evidence-based child injury prevention policies found New Zealand implemented only half of these interventional policies, again comparing poorly to comparative European OECD nations [5].

Children, although not traditionally thought of as part of the formal workforce in high income countries, do participate in work under less formal arrangements such as casual work during school holidays, part-time work after school, and work in family businesses. Additionally, they may be exposed to workplace hazards when they visit or live on worksites, such as farms. The only previous New Zealand study of child work-related fatal injury (WRFI) examined incidents from 1985 through 1998 [6]. This study reported child WRFI commonly occurred when children were bystanders to another person's work process or activity, with the agriculture sector and farms in particular the dominant setting for these injuries [6]. Studies on child WRFI in other countries are also limited, although available evidence from Australia and the United States show a similar pattern as New Zealand, with the agricultural sector being the most common industry involved in child WRFI [7–9].

Child fatal injuries are therefore rarely studied in a work-related context, despite work contributing significantly to the burden of unintentional injury for this age group and such child-related deaths being included in workplace safety legislative protections. Child WRFI data are difficult to obtain from official workplace injury notifications or injury compensation claims, as these databases typically only capture those aged 15 years and older. Furthermore, injuries sustained in a work setting are not readily identifiable in external cause codes as defined by the International Classification of Diseases (ICD) framework [10] and while some could be identified using corresponding ICD place of occurrence and activity codes higher levels of use of "other specified" or "unspecified" categories mean these are less readily utilized in research [11]. In contrast, in New Zealand, coronial records provide a complete and comprehensive source of child WRFI because all deaths that are 'sudden and unexpected' are referred to Coroners to determine the cause and circumstances of death. This study, utilizing Coronial records, provides the most up-to-date and comprehensive information available on child WRFI in New Zealand.

The research aims to address the current deficit in knowledge about child WRFI nationally and internationally, capturing all child fatalities where a work exposure directly or indirectly contributed to the causes and circumstances of the fatal injury incident. All children who were fatally injured on a worksite, in a public place or on a public road as a result of employment (paid, unpaid or in-kind for family business) or due to another person's work were included. This research will provide directions for preventive actions by using coronial case file data to establish a complete and comprehensive cohort of all WRFI in children from 1999 to 2014 in New Zealand.

2. Materials and Methods

Unintentional work-related fatal injuries of children aged less than 15 years were examined as part of a larger study of work-related injury fatalities in New Zealand [12,13]. In brief, potential WRFI cases with a date of death registration on or between 1 January 1999 and 31 December 2014 were identified using New Zealand's Mortality Collection, the most complete data source for all New Zealand deaths, including work-related injury fatalities. Injury deaths were identified in the Mortality Collection as those with an underlying cause of death coded to an external cause in the International Classification of Disease (ICD-10-AM) range V01 to X59, X85 to Y34, Y85 to 86, Y87.2, Y87.2 and Y89.9 [10]. Linkage to coronial records held by the National Coronial Information System was undertaken with all corresponding coronial records reviewed for work-relatedness. Coronial files were found for 98% of all 1335 relevant external cause deaths for children.

A broad definition of work-relatedness, compared with official data definitions, was used to capture all child fatalities to which a workplace exposure contributed. The work-relatedness of a fatal injury event was decided based on whether the decedent, at the time of the fatal incident, was: working for pay, profit or payment in kind; assisting with work in an unpaid capacity; was engaged in other work-related activities even when on a break or away from the workplace; or was a bystander (as defined below) to another person's work activity. All fatal injury cases determined to be work-related were broadly classified as one of the following.

Worker deaths: the decedent was fatally injured in the course of work duties in a workplace (referred to as workplace WRFI), or on a public road (referred to as work-traffic WRFI).

Bystander deaths: the decedent was not working but died as a result of someone else's work activity regardless of fault (referred to as bystander WRFI). These deaths could be further classified as bystander deaths occurring on a public road (work-traffic bystander), at a work place (workplace bystander) or to students of primary school age or older where the incident occurred during school time or while they were performing a task directly connected with their course (students).

Rural deaths: the decedent was fatally injured on a rural workplace (farm) where the circumstances did not satisfy the worker or bystander definitions above. This group includes farm deaths in children where it was difficult to ascertain the relative contribution of work and non-work exposures.

Socio-demographic characteristics including age, sex and ethnicity were obtained from the Mortality Collection. Prioritised ethnicity was determined by categorising individuals with multiple ethnicity responses in the order of Māori first, then Pacific, Asian and finally European/Other to provide a single response as per Ministry of Health ethnicity protocols [14]. Small area geographical meshblocks were coded from the physical address where the injury incident occurred. Small area-level deprivation was then derived using the 2013 New Zealand Deprivation Index (NZDep), with deciles categorised into quintiles, with '1–2' representing those living in the least and '9–10' the most deprived areas [15]. Mechanism of injury, location of injury incident, and agency and industry of incident were obtained from coronial records. Standard coding frameworks including the Type of Occurrence Classification System (TOOCS) and the Australian New Zealand Standard Industry Classification (ANZSIC) were used [16,17].

To describe the burden and patterns of child WRFI, frequencies and percentages were calculated. The risk of child WRFI was calculated by age group, sex, ethnicity and deprivation using incidence rates per 100,000 person years with 95% confidence intervals (95% CI). Population estimates for children aged less than 15 from the 2000, 2006 and 2013 Census were obtained from Statistics NZ with denominators for non-census years estimated by linear interpolation and extrapolation. Data were analysed using Stata V13.1 SE [18].

To illustrate the most common circumstances of child WRFI, a series of narrative "profiles" were created using a combination of quantitative data (analysis described above) and qualitative analyses. Qualitative analyses used a thematic analytical approach examining what the decedent was doing prior to the injury incident, what went wrong to cause the injury and the cause of death.

Ethical approval for this study was granted by the University of Otago Human Ethics Committee (Ref 15/065), the National Coronial Information System (Ref NZ007), and Health and Disability Ethics Committee (Ref OTA/99/02/008/AM05).

3. Results

3.1. Child Work-Related Fatal Injuries

Of the 1335 injury deaths of New Zealand children less than 15 years of age from 1999 through 2014, 206 (15%) were classified as being work-related. This equates to an average of 13 deaths per year, or 1.54 deaths per 100,000 children per year (Table 1). The overwhelming majority (91%) of these WRFI were bystanders to another person's work activity, with a slightly higher proportion of these fatalities occurring in workplaces (n = 93) compared with the work-traffic setting (n = 84). Of the few (n = 9) workers identified, one was aged 5–9 years and the remainder aged 10–14 years. A small number of deaths were children in rural workplaces.

3.2. Multiple Fatality Incidents

Among the 206 children who were fatally injured, 160 (78%) were involved in single fatality incidents, and 46 (22%) were involved in multiple fatality incidents, giving a total of 193 fatal incidents over the

16-year study period. Of the 46 multiple fatality incidents, 25 (54%) incidents included more than one child aged 0–14, primarily involving two child fatalities; however, one incident involved three.

Table 1. Work circumstance of work-related fatal injuries to children (0–14 years), New Zealand, 1999–2014.

Work Circumstances	Frequency n (%)	Rate (95% CI) per 100,000 Person Years
Working	9 (4.4)	0.06 (0.03–0.12)
Bystander	187 (90.7)	1.39 (1.21–1.61)
Rural workplace	10 (4.9)	0.07 (0.04–0.13)
Total	206 (100.0)	1.54 (1.34–1.77)

Abbreviations: Rate—incidence rate per 100,000 person years, 95% CI—95% Confidence Interval.

3.3. Socio-Demographic Characteristics

Regardless of work-related injury setting, it was more common for males (64%) to be fatally injured than females (36%), with the incidence of WRFI higher than that for females (1.9, 95% CI 1.5, 2.1 compared with 1.1, 95% CI 0.8, 1.3) (Table 2). The burden of child WRFI was split fairly evenly across the three age groups. Younger children aged 0–4 years were more commonly involved in workplace deaths (43%), while older children were slightly more likely to have sustained work injuries in the work-traffic setting (38% of 10–14 years). The incident rate was highest in 0–4 year-olds with 1.7 (95% CI 1.3, 2.1) deaths per 100,000 person years.

Table 2. Socio-demographic characteristics by location of injury, work-related fatalities to children (0–14 years), New Zealand, 1999–2014.

Characteristics	Work-Traffic n = 96 n (%)	Workplace n = 110 n (%)	Total n = 206 n (%)	Rate (95% CI) per 100,000 Person Years
Sex				
Male	57 (59.4)	75 (68.2)	132 (64.1)	1.93 (1.54–2.18)
Female	39 (40.6)	35 (31.8)	74 (35.9)	1.14 (0.83–1.33)
Age group				
0–4 years	28 (29.2)	47 (42.7)	75 (36.4)	1.71 (1.35–2.14)
5–9 years	32 (33.3)	31 (28.2)	63 (30.6)	1.42 (1.09–1.82)
10–14 years	35 (37.5)	33 (29.1)	68 (33.0)	1.49 (1.16–1.89)
Ethnicity				
European	44 (45.8)	69 (62.7)	113 (54.9)	1.60 (1.32–1.92)
Māori	35 (36.5)	30 (27.3)	65 (31.6)	1.96 (1.15–2.50)
Asian	7 (7.3)	7 (6.4)	14 (6.8)	1.13 (0.61–1.90)
Pacific	9 (9.4)	4 (3.6)	13 (6.3)	1.05 (0.55–1.79)
Other	1 (1.0)	0 (0.0)	1 (0.5)	0.17 (0.04–0.90)
NZDep Index				
1–2 (least deprived)	14 (14.5)	13 (11.8)	27 (13.1)	1.11 (0.72–1.16)
3–4	20 (20.8)	19 (17.2)	39 (18.9)	1.66 (1.18–2.26)
5–6	10 (10.4)	16 (24.5)	26 (12.6)	1.03 (0.67–1.50)
7–8	13 (13.5)	27 (24.5)	40 (19.4)	1.43 (1.02–1.94)
9–10 (most deprived)	38 (39.5)	26 (23.6)	64 (31.0)	1.97 (1.52–2.52)

Abbreviations: NZDep Index—New Zealand Deprivation Index, Rate—incidence rate per 100,000 person years, 95% CI—95% Confidence Interval.

The greatest number of child WRFI was observed in children of European ethnicity, followed by those of Māori ethnicity. However, the rate of child WRFI was highest amongst Māori children (1.9 per

100,00 person years, 95% CI 1.1, 2.5) followed by those of European ethnicity (1.6, 95% CI 1.3, 1.9) Among deaths of Māori children, most occurred in work-traffic settings, while among those of European ethnicity the majority of deaths occurred in the workplace. There were no clear differences observed by level of deprivation other than the rate for the most deprived group of children (NZ Dep 9–10) being the highest.

3.4. Incident and Injury Characteristics

Over one third of all child work-related injury deaths occurred in the major industry grouping of agriculture, forestry and fishing (37%), almost exclusively involving agriculture (Table 3). Agriculture was the largest single industry group across all child age groups, with the largest contribution occurring in children under five years of age (40%). One in five child WRFI involved the 'transport, postal and warehousing' major sector (20%), predominantly in the transport sector.

Table 3. Industry, location, activity and mechanism of work-related fatal injuries to children (0–14 years), New Zealand, 1999–2014.

Characteristics	0–4 Years n = 75 n (%)	5–9 Years n = 63 n (%)	10–14 Years n = 68 n (%)	Total n = 206 n (%)
Industry of incident				
Agriculture, forestry & fishing	30 (40.0)	23 (36.5)	23 (33.8)	76 (36.9)
Transport, postal & warehousing	16 (21.6)	14 (22.2)	13 (19.1)	43 (20.9)
Arts & recreation	12 (16.0)	5 (7.9)	3 (4.4)	20 (9.7)
Education & training	0 (0.0)	3 (4.8)	10 (14.7)	13 (6.3)
Construction	3 (4.0)	5 (7.9)	3 (4.4)	11 (5.3)
Other	14 (18.7)	13 (20.6)	16 (23.5)	43 (20.9)
Location				
Public road	24 (32.0)	32 (50.8)	36 (52.9)	92 (44.6)
Farm	30 (40.0)	20 (31.8)	21 (30.9)	71 (34.5)
Home	8 (10.7)	0 (0.0)	0 (0.0)	8 (3.9)
School	2 (2.7)	3 (4.8)	3 (4.4)	8 (3.9)
Recreation/sport	7 (9.3)	1 (1.6)	2 (2.9)	10 (4.9)
Industrial/construction	2 (2.7)	3 (4.8)	0 (0.0)	5 (2.4)
Unspecified/other	2 (2.7)	4 (6.3)	6 (8.9)	12 (5.8)
Urban-rural indicator				
Urban	30 (40.0)	31 (49.2)	32 (47.1)	93 (45.2)
Rural	45 (60.0)	32 (50.7)	36 (52.9)	113 (54.8)
Activity				
Passenger, in/on vehicle	26 (34.7)	26 (41.3)	19 (27.9)	71 (34.5)
Recreation/playing	30 (40.0)	14 (22.2)	11 (16.2)	55 (26.7)
Driving vehicle	1 (1.3)	7 (11.1)	13 (19.1)	21 (10.2)
Riding (horse, bicycle)	0 (0.0)	6 (9.5)	10 (14.7)	16 (7.8)
Helping out	2 (2.7)	2 (3.2)	3 (4.4)	7 (3.4)
Other	16 (21.3)	8 (12.7)	12 (17.6)	36 (17.5)
Mechanism				
Vehicle crash	21 (28.0)	26 (41.3)	24 (35.3)	71 (34.5)
Hit by moving object	27 (36.0)	20 (31.8)	20 (29.4)	67 (32.5)
Electricity, drowning	17 (22.7)	7 (11.1)	8 (11.8)	32 (15.5)
Vehicle rollover	4 (5.3)	6 (9.5)	9 (13.2)	19 (9.2)
Other and multiple	6 (8.0)	4 (6.4)	7 (9.3)	17 (8.3)

The most common incident locations of child WRFI were public roads (45%) and farms (35%). For those under five years of age, WRFI were more commonly sustained on farms (40%) while children aged 5–14 years were more likely to be fatally injured on public roads (51% in 5–9 years, 53% in 10–14 years). Fatalities occurring in industrial/construction settings were rare. Of the 71 children who sustained WRFI on farms, the majority normally resided on the farm where the incident occurred or in surrounding rural areas ($n = 59$, 83%). Children fatally injured while visiting farms were older (> 5 years) and most commonly operating farm vehicles, such as quad bikes.

Overall, the most common activities at the time of the WRFI were being transported as a passenger in, or on, a vehicle (34%), followed by recreation/playing (26%). It was more common for children under five years of age to be fatally injured while engaged in recreation/playing (40%) activities than it was for older children. Almost 20% of older children (10–14 years) were fatally injured while driving vehicles.

The mechanism of injury most commonly involved in child WRFI was vehicle crashes (34%) and being hit by moving objects (32%) with these incidents occurring on- or off-road. Slightly more children under five years of age were fatally injured when hit by a moving object compared with vehicle crashes, while the opposite pattern was observed for older children.

3.5. Agency

The breakdown agent, which is the agent immediately triggering the fatal injury incident, was most commonly human behavior (39%) (Table 4). Over half of child WRFI in those aged 0–4 years involved human behavior: particularly the child's own behavior, such as a being attracted to an agricultural pond but with, presumably, little cognitive awareness of the hazard presented by water; and preoccupied caregivers, such as working parents distracted by a work activity while supervising young children. The next most common breakdown agent was vehicles (31%), particularly involving cars and utility vehicles. Vehicles were the most common trigger for fatal incidents involving children aged 5–9 years (41%) and those aged 10–14 years (32%). Environmental factors were most common amongst children aged 10–14 years, frequently including sloping or rough ground surfaces which contributes to loss of control of a vehicle, such as a quad bike on a farm.

Table 4. Agency triggering the work-related incident (breakdown agent), among children (0–14 years), New Zealand, 1999–2014.

Characteristics	0–4 Years $n = 75$ n (%)	5–9 Years $n = 63$ n (%)	10–14 Years $n = 68$ n (%)	Total n (%)
Vehicle	15 (20.0)	26 (41.2)	22 (32.3)	63 (30.5)
Animal/Human behavior	41 (54.6)	24 (38.0)	16 (23.5)	81 (39.3)
Environment	10 (13.3)	7 (11.1)	18 (26.4)	35 (16.9)
Manufactured material	1 (1.3)	4 (6.3)	3 (4.4)	8 (3.8)
Machinery/tools	6 (8.0)	2 (3.1)	6 (8.8)	14 (6.7)
Other/unspecified	2 (2.6)	0	3 (4.4)	5 (2.4)

3.6. Narratives of Common Circumstances

The majority of child WRFI incidents involved one of four narratives representing the most common and recurrent circumstances of fatal injury: 1) unsupervised young children on farms; 2) children operating a vehicle on farms; 3) children as vehicle passengers involved in a collision with a working vehicle; and 4) children hit as a pedestrian or cyclist by a working vehicle.

The first scenario includes distracted supervision of young children on farms. In this scenario, young children were often playing unsupervised in a secure area around a farm house or while accompanying working parents on the farm. The young child was able to leave the "supervised area", a space often considered to be secure by the parent. The young child was attracted to a water feature, such as a stream or an unfenced agricultural pond, or towards animals, and was fatally injured. There was often a delay before the child is noticed missing, which points to the supervising parents having a high level of trust in the security of the space they place their child within and the difficulties in maintaining focus on child safety while engaged in work activities.

Another common scenario was children operating adult-sized quad bikes on a farm for the common purpose of rounding up cows or other animals, or engaging in a farm-related recreational activity. In these situations, the child lost control of the quad bike while operating the quad bike. The cause of the loss of control was often due to an unexpected change in terrain or due to loss of traction on a sloping paddock. In all cases, the quad bike has flipped landing on top of the child, inflicting crush injuries. The child was generally unaccompanied by an adult and is found dead at the scene.

Working vehicles on public roads is also a common scenario involving child WRFI. The most common road-bystander scenarios involved children as passengers in a non-working vehicle where, in many cases, an adult driver made an error, such as a dangerous overtaking manoeuvre or crossing the dividing centre lines on a two-way road. The non-working vehicle invariably collided head on with an oncoming working vehicle, most commonly a heavy truck, resulting in substantial impact injuries in all occupants of the non-working vehicle. Another further common scenario involves children as pedestrians at intersections or crossing the road, or as a cyclist on public roads, being struck by a working vehicle. Often, the working vehicle in this scenario was a large truck where the child was located within the blind spot of the truck's mirrors resulting in the driver being unaware of the presence of the child prior to the incident.

4. Discussion

Work-related fatal injury contributes substantially to the total burden of unintentional fatal injury in New Zealand; 15% of the total burden of fatal unintentional injury in children in New Zealand during the period 1999–2014 was attributable to a work exposure. Both the former Health and Safety in Employment Amendment Act 2002 and the new Health and Safety at Work Act 2015 require employers and the responsible Government Agencies to protect all people who come into contact with workplaces, including children [19,20]. As such, there is a clear legislative mandate to prevent WRFI in children and investigate the circumstances of any that do occur. This study's findings indicate the highest risks for child WRFI are in males, those under five years of age and those of Māori or European ethnicity. Child WRFI most commonly involved vehicle crashes or being hit by moving objects in incidents occurring on farms or public road. The main industries involved included the agriculture and transport sector.

This is a largely hidden burden as New Zealand's official WRFI data excludes bystander deaths, thereby excluding most WRFI deaths in children. This study's novel data therefore lead to the identification of important missed opportunities to reduce the broader public health impact of work-related fatalities in New Zealand. Updated accurate data on the current patterns of work-related fatalities inform where workplace interventions to prevent fatalities to children are needed and allows for the monitoring in trends in child WRFI over time. Combined with previously published child WRFI data, this study has demonstrated a declining trend in child WRFI between periods. This study identified 1.5 (95% CI 1.3, 1.7) work-related fatal injuries per 100,000 children for the period 1999 to 2014, a considerable decrease compared to the rate of 2.1 (95% CI 1.8, 2.4) in the study that covered from 1985–1998 [6]. However, despite the decline, similar patterns of child WRFI to those described earlier remain: bystander deaths dominate and the agricultural industry is the most common industry in which child WRFI occurs [8]. While there was an overall decline in rates of WRFI in adult workers in New Zealand over a similar period, these trends have been variable [21]. For example, adult workers in the primary production sector of agriculture, forestry and fisheries experienced an increase in fatal injury risk over this time [21].

The majority of children who sustained WRFI were bystanders, consistent with patterns of work involvement observed in children in Australia [7,9] and, as would be expected, given the low proportion of children engaged in formal or informal work, especially at a young age. The preponderance of bystander deaths in children reflects inadequate control over the hazards generated by work activities largely under the direct control of an adult worker, thus providing insight into the failures in the control of hazards in these work situations. This study found it was rare for children less than 15 years to be fatally injured as a worker. The circumstances of work involvement change with increasing age. As children get older and their physical and cognitive abilities develop, there is increasing movement into the formal workforce which changes the exposure of the child to workplace hazards, and the pattern of fatalities becomes more like that of adults [21].

The age-related patterns of WRFI observed in this study are consistent with those observed elsewhere. The exposure of children to work hazards, even at a very young age, are partially explained by the norms and attitudes of parents. For example, children residing on New Zealand farms often accompany working parents, or are engaged in farm work, where there are distinctive patterns of exposure to farm tasks by age [22]. Families residing on farms can perceive that children raised on farms are more aware of hazards and are more capable of handling risky agricultural tasks even at a young age [23]. North American Guidelines informing adults of agricultural tasks appropriate to the different child physical and cognitive developmental stages and corresponding abilities of children have been shown to be effective at reducing the burden of injury in children on farms [24].

Males are commonly over-represented in child WRFI, particularly on farms [9]. Gendered patterns of exposure to work hazards occur on New Zealand farms, with male children more involved in farm tasks involving machinery and vehicles resulting in increased risk of WRFI for males [22]. Māori children are over-represented in unintentional fatal injury, accounting for half of all child unintentional injury deaths in New Zealand [25]. This study's findings suggest injury prevention efforts to reduce child WRFI for Māori need to focus on reducing work-traffic crashes. Whilst child WRFI rates varied by level of deprivation, with the highest rate of child WRFI observed for the most deprived children, there were few other clear patterns observed. This is in contrast to the common trend of a gradient of risk of fatal injury with increasing levels of deprivation in child unintentional injury mortality overall in New Zealand [26]. Few other studies have considered this as a potential determinant of child WRFI.

Rural environments are an important determinant of child WRFI. The agricultural sector is consistently identified as being one of the highest risk groups for fatal injury in adult workers in New Zealand [27–29]. Others have previously identified children living on farms or rurally as carrying higher injury risks compared to other non-farming or urban counterparts [7,9,30,31]. In agriculture, unlike other industries, children provide informal labor for family farm operations at an early age and farms typically have dual purposes, being both a place of work and of residence. This poses higher risk of work-related injury for children residing on, or visiting farms, because they are exposed to common and high-risk hazards, such as farm machinery and moving vehicles [22], to which other children are not exposed.

Very young children are particularly vulnerable to WRFI on farms where high levels of active supervision are needed to keep them safe in a high hazard work environment. While a 2007/08 survey of NZ farms found it was uncommon for young children to accompany working adults on farms [22], when it does occur, it poses a particularly high risk of WRFI for young children. A lack of childcare options for rural farming families, and rural attitudes of including children in informal family farm work from a young age, have also been identified as a barrier to protecting farm children from the hazards of work [32]. Many farming parents in New Zealand feel that, in order to prevent injuries on farms, a child's access to active farming areas, as well to farm machinery or vehicles, should be restricted, or at a minimum properly supervised by an adult [22]. Other opportunities for prevention include the use of the most suitable vehicle to transport children on farms and the use of child restraints, such as seat belts and car seats in work vehicles to ensure the safety of children as occupants in vehicles used on- or off-road [33].

Other work contexts were also identified as being of concern. This study identified that work exposures make a substantive contribution to 28% of the total burden of transport-related fatalities involving children aged under 15 in New Zealand. Using public roads is a necessary part of everyday life for children; therefore, it is unsurprising that motor vehicle traffic crashes (MVTC) are the overall leading cause of death in New Zealand children aged less than 15, accounting for over a quarter of all child deaths for the period 2006–2010 [34]. While our finding highlights the potential for reducing child fatalities on public roads through the influence of workplace safety policy, few of these incidents were triggered by a work vehicle, which limits the possibilities for prevention through work safety actions. One area of direct influence of work, however, that needs to improve is heavy vehicle driver awareness of cyclists and pedestrians. To help with these sensory technologies, alerting drivers of the presence of cyclists or pedestrians in blind spots should be adopted on working vehicles. The implementation of other evidence-based traffic safety interventions, such as proper child car restraints, use of seatbelts, alcohol controls, and improved road infrastructure, such as physically divided roads on routes carrying high volumes of heavy working vehicles, provide other opportunities to reduce the burden of child WRFI [35]. However, it is really only the last of these that is primarily a work-related prevention initiative. Fatalities occurring in industrial or construction settings that are more common amongst working adults [21] were rare in children.

It is important that children's needs for preventive actions in the workplace are assessed alongside those of the working adult population because the patterns of child WRFI differ from those of adults. Simply applying injury interventions intended for adults may not adequately protect children. Children are considered vulnerable to WRFI due to their lack of power in the work organizational hierarchy, and their lack of physical and cognitive development, leading to children and adults underestimating risk [32]. Effective or promising strategies for preventing child injury broadly includes (listed from most to least effective) legislation, modification of the environment or a product, the use of safety devices, educational home visits, community based interventions and education and skills development [33,34].

New Zealand performs poorly in the prevention of child and adolescent fatal injury, with rates of child injury mortality ranking the worst out of out of 24 OECD countries [4]. A wide-ranging national strategy for child safety more broadly is currently lacking, with previous national strategic efforts, most notably the New Zealand Injury Prevention Strategy (operational from 2003 to 2013), falling victim to changes in political focus [36]. The Well Child/Tamariki Ora programme, which takes an integrated child health and development approach to improve child health and well-being, includes child safety. However, it predominantly targets home and transport-based injury risks [37]. Children are a notable omission from New Zealand's Health and Safety at Work Strategy despite the strategy's vision of "work [that] is healthy and safe for everyone in New Zealand" [38]. This situation serves to illustrate the lack of implementation of important and effective policy and legislative actions to improve safety for children [5]. Our study highlights the need for child safety strategies to address the substantial role of work exposures in addressing the burden of fatal injury for children in New Zealand. National strategies for farm safety have been developed in Australia; for example, farm focused interventions and education programmes have been implemented to address child safety issues on farms [39].

Overall, these findings identify where improvements in prevention efforts are needed to address child WRFI, serving to highlight the importance of managing work-related risks for children, particularly in the Agricultural sector. Most child WRFI are highly preventable, largely by adult intervention and enforcement of current workplace health and safety legislation. Furthermore, the recurrent common narrative scenarios point to the highly repetitive circumstances surrounding these incidents, implying that it is common to fail to learn from previous fatal incidents involving children. Interventions to address WRFI in the youngest children (0–4 years) should focus on improved adult supervision of children during play on farms, while interventions for children aged 5–14 years should focus on reducing vehicle crashes on public roads, alongside farm settings. To identify and address the hidden burden of child WRFI official data capturing work-related injuries should be expanded to capture fatal and non-fatal injuries sustained by children. Regular surveillance of the burden and patterns of child WRFI will directly inform interventions to change work practices harmful to children and allow for these incidents to be included in health and safety enforcement practice.

The availability of detail-rich Coronial records allowed for the comprehensive and accurate determination of work-relatedness and the collection of new information on the causes and circumstances of child WRFI unavailable from other data sources. The mandated requirement for all sudden and unexpected deaths to be notified to a Coroner for investigation means that virtually all child deaths due to external causes receive an inquest to determine the cause and circumstance of the fatal injury providing a comprehensive population basis for informing directions for intervention. The inclusion of common narratives capturing the recurring circumstances of injury is novel for studies describing the burden of child fatalities. This study is limited to 2014 as the most recent year available due to the lengthy time it takes for a Coronial inquest to be "closed" and become available for research purposes, limiting the currency of the data. It is a strength that this study expands the range of childhood work-related deaths to consider all industry groups with many previous studies focusing only on fatalities occurring on farms. This study is limited to fatal injury in children and the mortality rates for children fatally injured while working used the total child population due to the lack of working population denominators for children. The inclusion of traffic fatalities where the working vehicle was not "at fault" limits the generalisability to other countries with "at-fault" systems restricted to cases where there was liability on the part of a working vehicle. However, inclusion of cases regardless of fault in this study is consistent with New Zealand's no-fault universal accident compensation system.

5. Conclusions

This study found that work makes a notable contribution to the total burden of fatal injury in children. Most child WRFI are highly preventable, largely by adult intervention and enforcement of workplace health and safety legislation. Greater attention on managing work-related risks for children, particularly in rural farm and transport settings, would result in a significant reduction in the injury mortality rates of New Zealand children.

Author Contributions: Conceptualization, R.L., B.M., G.D. and T.D.; methodology, R.L., B.M., G.D., B.d.G., and T.D.; data management, B.d.G.; formal analysis, R.L.; investigation, B.M.; resources, B.d.G., B.M.; data curation, B.d.G.; writing—original draft preparation, R.L.; writing review and editing, G.D., B.M., T.D.; project administration, B.M., B.d.G.; funding acquisition, R.L. All authors have read and agreed to the published version of the manuscript.

Funding: This research was funded by a 2018 University of Otago Research Grant.

Institutional Review Board Statement: The study was conducted according to the guidelines of the Declaration of Helsinki, and approved by the the University of Otago Human Ethics Committee (Ref 15/065), the National Coronial Information System (Ref NZ007), and Health and Disability Ethics Committee (Ref OTA/99/02/008/AM05).

Informed Consent Statement: Not applicable—all participants were deceased.

Data Availability Statement: Data were obtained from a secondary provider and are not publicly available.

Acknowledgments: The authors are grateful to staff from Archives NZ, Coronial Services—Tribunals Division at Ministry of Justice and the National Coronial Information Service in Australia for the provision of coronial files. We acknowledge our research assistants (Rose Moffat and Sarah Peters) for their careful review and coding of coronial files. We would also like to acknowledge the University of Otago—Statistics New Zealand Consort Agreement and Glenda

Oben, New Zealand Child and Youth Epidemiology Service, University of Otago for the provision of denominators. We are grateful for the earlier data preparation and analyses undertaken by Louise Thorn.

Conflicts of Interest: The authors declare no conflict of interest.

References

1. Ministry of Health and Accident Compensation Corporation. *Injury-Related Health Loss: A Report from the New Zealand Burden of Disease, Injuries and Risk Factors Study 2006–2016*; Ministry of Health: Wellington, New Zealand, 2013.
2. Craig, E.; Jackson, C.; Han, D.Y.; NZCYES Steering Committee. *Monitoring the Health of New Zealand Children and Young People: Indicator Handbook*; Paediatric Society & New Zealand Child and Youth Epidemiology Service: Auckland, New Zealand, 2007.
3. Shaw, C.; Blakely, T.; Crampton, P.; Aitkinson, J. The contribution of causes of death to socioeconomic inequalities in child mortality: New Zealand 1981–1999. *N. Z. Med. J.* **2005**, *118*, e1779.
4. United Nations International Children's Emergency Fund (UNICEF). *Child Poverty in Perspective: An Overview of Child Well-Being in Rich Countries*; UNICEF Innocenti Research Centre: Florence, Italy, 2007.
5. Shepherd, M.; Kool, B.; Ameratunga, S.; Bland, V.; Hassall, I.; Chambers, J.; Carter, W.; Dalziel, S. Preventing child unintentional injury deaths: Prioritising the response to the New Zealand Child and Adolescent Injury Report Card. *Aus. N. Z. J. Public Health* **2013**, *37*, 470–474. [CrossRef] [PubMed]
6. Lilley, R.; Feyer, A.-M.; Langley, J.; Wren, J. The New Zealand child work-related fatal injury study: 1985–1998. *N. Z. Med. J.* **2004**, *117*, U 1194.
7. Mandryk, J.; Harrison, J. Work-related deaths of children and adolescents in Australia, 1982 to 1984. *Aus. J. Public Health* **1995**, *19*, 46–49. [CrossRef] [PubMed]
8. Fassa, A.G. Illustrative example A: Work-related injuries. In *Child Labour: A Public Health Perspective*; Fassa, A.G., Parker, D.L., Scanlon, T.J., Eds.; Oxford University Press: New York, NY, USA, 2010.
9. Mitchell, R.J.; Franklin, R.C.; Driscoll, T.R. Farm-related fatalities involving children in Australia, 1989–92. *Aus. N. Z. J. Public Health* **2001**, *25*, 307–314. [CrossRef] [PubMed]
10. World Health Organization. *ICD-10: International Statistical Classification of Diseases and Related Health Problems: Tenth Revision*, 2nd ed.; World Health Organization: Geneva, Switzerland, 2004.
11. Langley, J.; Davie, G.; Simpson, J. Quality of hospital discharge data for injury prevention. *Inj. Prev.* **2007**, *13*, 42–44. [CrossRef] [PubMed]
12. Lilley, R.; Maclennan, B.; McNoe, B.; Davie, G.; Horsburgh, S.; Driscoll, T. A decade of fatal injuries in workers in New Zealand: Insights from a comprehensive national observational study. *Inj. Prev.* **2020**. [CrossRef] [PubMed]
13. Lilley, R.; McNoe, B.; Davie, G.; Horsburgh, S.; Maclennan, B.; Driscoll, T. Identifying opportunities to prevent work-related fatal injury in New Zealand using 40 years of coronial records: Protocol for a retrospective case review study. *Inj. Epidemiol.* **2019**, *6*, 16. [CrossRef] [PubMed]
14. Ministry of Health. *HISO 10001:2017 Ethnicity Data Protocols*; Ministry of Health: Wellington, New Zealand, 2017.
15. Atkinson, J.; Salmond, C.; Crampton, P. *NZDep2013 Index of Deprivation*; University of Otago: Wellington, New Zealand, 2014.
16. National Occupational Health and Safety Commission. *Type of Occurrence Classification System*; Australian Government Publishing Service: Canberra, Australia, 1990.
17. Statistics New Zealand. *Australia New Zealand Standard Industrial Classification 2006 V1.0.0*; 2006. Available online: http://aria.stats.govt.nz (accessed on 10 October 2020).
18. StataCorp. *Stata Statistical Software: Release 13*; StataCorp LP: College Stations, TX, USA, 2013.
19. New Zealand Government. *Health and Safety in Employment Amendment Act 2002*; New Zealand Government: Wellington, New Zealand, 2002.
20. New Zealand Government. *Health and Safety at Work Act 2015*; New Zealand Government: Wellington, New Zealand, 2015.

21. Lilley, R.; Maclennan, B.; Davie, G.; McNoe, B.; Horsburgh, S.; Driscoll, T. Decade of variable progress: Trends in fatal injury in workers in New Zeaalnd from a national observational study. *Occup. Environ. Med.* **2020**. Epub ahead of print [26 October 2020]. [CrossRef] [PubMed]
22. Cryer, C.; Lovelock, K.; Lilley, R. *Effective Occupational Health Interventions in Agriculture. A Report of a Survey of Risk Factors and Exposures on Farms*; Injury Prevention Research Unit: Dunedin, New Zealand, 2009.
23. Neufeld, S.; Wright, S.M.; Gaut, J. Not raising a bubble kid: Farm parents' attitudes and practices regarding the employment, training and supervision of their children. *J. Rural Health* **2002**, *18*, 57–66. [CrossRef] [PubMed]
24. Gadomski, A.; Ackerman, S.P.; Jenkins, P. Efficacy of the North American Guidelines for Children's Agricultural Tasks in reducing childhood agricultural injuries. *Am. J. Public Health* **2006**, *96*, 22–27. [CrossRef] [PubMed]
25. Safekids, A. *Tamariki Māori Unintentional Injuries*; Safekids Aotearoa: Auckland, New Zealand, 2017.
26. Shaw, C. *Socioeconomic Gradients in Child Mortality: New Zealand 1981–1999*; University of Otago: Dunedin, New Zealand, 2004.
27. Horsburgh, S.; Feyer, A.-M.; Langley, J. Fatal work-related injuries in agriculture production and service to agriculture sectors of New Zealand, 1985–94. *Occup. Environ. Med.* **2001**, *58*, 489–495. [CrossRef] [PubMed]
28. Cryer, C.; Fleming, C. A review of work-related fatal injuries in New Zealand 1975–84—numbers, rates and trends. *N. Z. Med. J.* **1987**, *100*, 1–6. [PubMed]
29. Feyer, A.-M.; Langley, J.; Howard, M.; Horsburgh, S.; Wright, C.; Alsop, J.; Cryer, C. The work-related fatal injury study: Numbers, rates and trends of work-related fatal injuries in New Zealand 1985–1994. *N. Z. Med. J.* **2001**, *114*, 6. [PubMed]
30. Kim, K.; Ozegovic, D.; Voaklander, D.C. Differences in incidence of injury between rural and urban children in Canada and the USA: A systematic review. *Inj. Prev.* **2012**, *18*, 264–271. [CrossRef] [PubMed]
31. Peachey, K.-L.; Lower, T.; Rolfe, M. Protecting the future: Fatal incidents on Australian farms involving children (2001–2019). *Aus. J. Rural Health* **2020**. [CrossRef] [PubMed]
32. Wright, S.M.; Marlenga, B.; Lee, B.C. Childhood agricultural injuries: An update for clinicians. *Current Probl. Pediatr. Adolesc. Health Care* **2013**, *43*, 20–44. [CrossRef] [PubMed]
33. Fragar, L.; Gibson, C.; Hendrerson, A.; Franklin, R. *Farmsafe Farms for Kids. Evidence Based Solutions for Child Injury on Australian Farms*; Australian Cetnre for Agricultural Health and Safety: Moree, Australia, 2003.
34. Safekids, A. *Child Unintentional Deaths and Injuries in New Zealand, and Prevention Strategies*; Safekids Aotearoa: Auckland, New Zealand, 2015.
35. McMahon, K.; Gopalakrishna, G.; Stevenson, M. Chapter 2. Road traffic injuries. In *World Report on Child Injury Prevention*; Peden, M., Oyegbite, K., Ozanne-Smith, J., Hyder, A.A., Branche, C., Rahman, A.K.M.F., Rivara, F., Bartolomeos, K., Eds.; World Health Organization: Geneva, Switzerland, 2008.
36. Smeh, D.; Bonokoski, N. New Zealand Injury Prevention Strategy. In *Casebook of Traumatic Injury Prevention*; Volpe, R., Ed.; Springer: Cham, Switzerland, 2020.
37. Ministry of Health. *The Well Child/Tamariki Ora Programme*; 2020. Available online: www.wellchild.org.nz (accessed on 10 October 2020).
38. New Zealand Government. *Health and Safety at Work Strategy. 2018–2028*; New Zealand Government: Wellington, New Zealand, 2018.
39. Farmsafe Australia. *Child Safety on Farms: A Framework for a National Strategy in Australia*; Farmsafe Australia: Moree, Australia, 1999.

Publisher's Note: MDPI stays neutral with regard to jurisdictional claims in published maps and institutional affiliations.

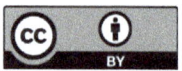

© 2020 by the authors. Licensee MDPI, Basel, Switzerland. This article is an open access article distributed under the terms and conditions of the Creative Commons Attribution (CC BY) license (http://creativecommons.org/licenses/by/4.0/).

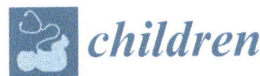

Article

The Correlation between Oral Self-Harm and Ethnicity in Institutionalized Children

Alexandra Mihaela Stoica [1], Oana Elena Stoica [2], Ramona Elena Vlad [1], Anca Maria Pop [3,*] and Monica Monea [1]

[1] Department of Odontology and Oral Pathology, George Emil Palade University of Medicine, Pharmacy, Science, and Technology of Târgu Mureș, 540139 Târgu Mureș, Romania; alexandra.stoica@umfst.ro (A.M.S.); ramona.vlad@umfst.ro (R.E.V.); monica.monea@umfst.ro (M.M.)
[2] Department of Pedodontics, George Emil Palade University of Medicine, Pharmacy, Science, and Technology of Târgu Mureș, 540139 Târgu Mureș, Romania; oana.stoica@umfst.ro
[3] Faculty of Medicine, George Emil Palade University of Medicine, Pharmacy, Science, and Technology of Târgu Mureș, 540139 Târgu Mureș, Romania
* Correspondence: ancapop98@yahoo.com

Received: 15 November 2020; Accepted: 21 December 2020; Published: 23 December 2020

Abstract: Oral self-harm was described in institutionalized children who share a lack of emotional attention; frequently these children experience feelings such as neglect, loneliness, isolation or lack of connection with the world. The aim of our paper was to conduct a cross-sectional study in order to assess the prevalence of this behavior and its correlation with ethnicity among children from three institutions located in the central part of Romania. We examined 116 children from three ethnic groups, Romanians, Hungarians and local Roma population aged between 10–14 years old. The oral soft tissues were evaluated by one dentist who recorded the lesions of lips, buccal mucosa, commissures and tongue; data were statistically analyzed at a level of significance of $p < 0.05$. We found oral self-harm lesions in 18.1% participants, with statistically significant higher odds in girls ($p = 0.03$). The results showed an association between ethnicity and the development of these lesions (Chi-square $p = 0.04$). The most frequent lesions were located at oral commissures (35.48%), buccal mucosa (29.03%) and upper lip (19.36%). Oral self-harm lesions have a high incidence among institutionalized children in Romania. Identification of these cases in early stages is important, as these conditions are known to be aggravated during adolescence and adulthood.

Keywords: self-injurious behavior; institutionalized child; oral manifestations

1. Introduction

Self-mutilation is defined as a behavioral disturbance that consists of self-induced damage to body tissues, which might be associated in some cases with a conscious intent to commit suicide. Also called self-harm, it includes any intentional injury to one's own body [1–4]. Historically, the first institutions for abandoned children can be traced back in Europe since the Middle Ages; they came into prominence in the 19th century in Western Europe, today being common in different parts of the world such as Asia, Central and South America, the Middle East or Africa. In the United States, orphanages were documented in the first half of the 20th century [5].

At present, worldwide there are between 8–10 million children living in different types of institution [6] and there is much scientific evidence that their psychological development is impaired by these life conditions [7]; furthermore, the trend of placing children in institutions appears to be growing [8,9]. According to data from literature, institutional care in Romania was associated with an impairment of the physical development [10] and also children who spent more than 6 months in an institution had higher rates of autism symptoms, inattention or disinhibited social engagement [11]. Due to the demands of taking care of a large number of children, the caregivers rarely interact with children in a warm manner, as their activity is frequently limited to routine care, such as feeding or toileting [12]. Therefore, most institutionalized children experience poor caregiver-child interaction and their physical, cognitive and social development is often delayed. Moreover, scientific data showed that these results are caused mainly by the quality of caregiver-child relationships, rather than by the quality of medical care and nutrition [13]. The inability to live with their parents predisposes institutionalized children to low self-esteem and impaired psychosocial development (attention problems or lower intelligence quotient) [7], which might represent confounding factors in the analysis of the correlation between self-harm and institutionalization.

In institutionalized children, the relief of emotional pain could be expressed by self-harm, as the physical wounds they create on themselves is a sign of their emotional suffering [14]. The self-harm behavior has many causes, including stressful life events or mental disorders such as depression or anxiety [15]. Adolescents use deliberate self-harm methods such as cutting, poisoning or overdosing, while children usually scratch or bite themselves; this phenomenon may start during childhood and intensifies in adolescents and young adults, girls being considered more vulnerable to this behavior than boys [16]. Among the etiological factors of deliberate self-harm the following conditions were included: depression, low self-esteem and sense of persistent hopelessness, attempts to seek help from others, poverty, abuse, attempts to resist suicidal thoughts and family dysfunction. The early detection of non-suicidal self-injury (NSSI) allows immediate intervention which might help these children stop this behavior. Left undiagnosed for a long period of time, NSSI becomes more frequent, severe and versatile, with negative consequences on the quality of life and more difficult recovery [17].

Oral self-harm (OSH) in institutionalized children occurs in connection with emotional, behavioral or even organic disorders. To date, most of the information comes from case series presentations and there are little scientific data regarding the frequency of OSH among abandoned children without mental disorders or retardation. Therefore, the aim of our paper was to conduct a cross-sectional study in order to assess the frequency and type of OSH among institutionalized children from three Romanian state centers. The null hypothesis to be tested was that there is no statistically significant difference regarding the prevalence of oral self-inflicted lesions, according to gender and ethnicity in children at puberty.

2. Materials and Methods

2.1. Study Design and Participants

Our investigation was conducted between December 2019–February 2020 in the Clinic of Odontology and Oral Pathology from the George Emil Palade University of Medicine, Pharmacy, Science, and Technology of Târgu Mureș, where there is a special program dedicated to dental medical care for institutionalized children, belonging to three state centers. The investigation was carried out after the approval obtained from the Ethics Committee of our university (No. 520/21.11.2019), accompanied by a written consent for the use of personal data signed in each case by the legal representative of the child (institution manager or legal guardian). Prior to enrolment in the study, children were also asked if they agreed to participate. We are located in the historical province of Transylvania, characterized by a multicultural and multiethnic population, represented mainly by Romanians, Hungarians and regional Roma. In order to address a source of bias related to the number of participants from each ethnicity, we decided to include close numbers in each group, according to age and gender. Moreover, all clinical examinations were carried out by one experienced dentist and data were recorded by one dental specialist. In our study we included 116 children aged between 10–14 years old, selected from a total of 167 children, based on application of inclusion criteria (status of institutionalized child for more than 5 years, age 10–14 years) and exclusion criteria (history of psychological counseling or psychiatric treatment, recordings of drugs or alcohol abuse, children with diagnosed neurologic or psychiatric disorders, known to be etiological factors of self-harm behavior, such as epilepsy, depression, anxiety or autism spectrum disorder) (Figure 1).

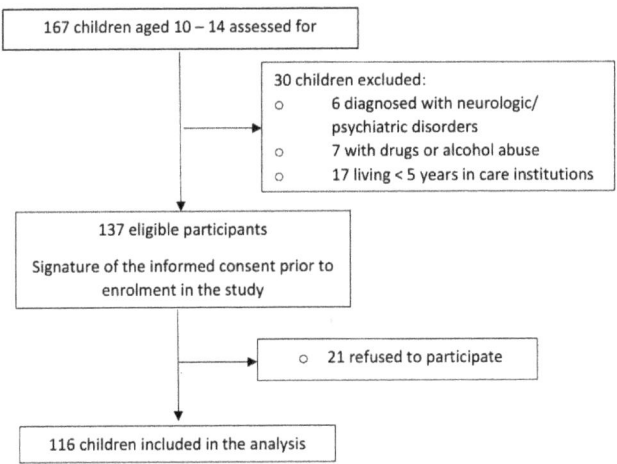

Figure 1. Flow diagram illustrating selection of participants to the study.

2.2. Clinical and Histopathological Examination

Ordinary dental examinations, with an emphasis on the health status of the lips, buccal mucosa and tongue (ulcerations, color change, surface aspect), were performed. In order to detect any changes from normal texture, the area between oral commissures was carefully evaluated by palpation. Cases in which a chronic evolution was suspected, resembling premalignant lesions, were further investigated by exfoliative cytology, using Papanicolau stain. All children who presented OSH were further referred to interdisciplinary evaluation by a psychologist and dental specialist.

2.3. Statistical Analysis

Statistical analysis was carried out using GraphPad Prism 7 for Windows (GraphPad Software, San Diego, CA, USA), by Fisher's exact test and Chi-square test. The continuous variables were expressed as mean ± standard deviation and categorical variables as percentages and frequency distribution. The level of statistical significance was set at a p value < 0.05 (two-tailed).

3. Results

The distribution of the study group based on gender and ethnicity is presented in Table 1.

Table 1. Distribution of the study group according to gender and ethnicity.

Gender/Ethnicity	Romanians	Hungarians	Roma	Total
Female	20 (17.24%)	19 (16.38%)	24 (20.69%)	63 (54.31%)
Male	17 (14.65%)	15 (12.93%)	21 (18.11%)	53 (45.69%)
Total	37 (31.89%)	34 (29.31%)	45 (38.8%)	116 (100%)

The mean age of the study group was 12.11 ± 1.36 years.

The presence of OSH was noticed in 21 participants (18.1%). According to Fisher's exact test, girls had statistically significant higher odds of presenting OSH than boys (odds ratio (OR) = 3.268, 95% confidence interval (CI): 1.108–9.643, $p = 0.03$) (Table 2).

Table 2. The distribution of lesions according to gender.

Gender/Oral Lesion	Oral Lesion Present	Oral Lesion Absent	Total
Female	16 (13.79%)	47 (40.52%)	63 (54.31%)
Male	5 (4.31%)	48 (41.38%)	53 (45.69%)
Total	21 (18.1%)	95 (81.9%)	116 (100%)

The results of our study showed that the presence of self-inflicted oral lesions is influenced by ethnicity (Chi-square original $p = 0.04$). After applying the Bonferroni correction, the level of statistical significance was adjusted at $p < 0.0167$. Therefore, Romanians had statistically significant lower odds of developing oral self-injuries compared to Roma participants (OR = 0.15, 95% CI: 0.03–0.75, $p = 0.0164$), but there was no significant difference neither between Romanians and Hungarians (OR = 0.22, 95% CI: 0.04–1.148, $p = 0.07$), nor between Hungarians and Roma participants (OR = 0.71, 95% CI: 0.24–2.06, $p = 0.6$) (Table 3).

Table 3. The distribution of oral lesions according to ethnicity.

Ethnicity/Oral Lesion	Oral Lesion Present	Oral Lesion Absent	Total
Romanian	2 (1.72%)	35 (30.17%)	37 (31.89%)
Hungarian	7 (6.03%)	27 (23.28%)	34 (29.31%)
Roma	12 (10.35%)	33 (28.45%)	45 (38.8%)
Total	21 (18.1%)	95 (81.9%)	116 (100%)

In Table 4 the types of encountered lesions are summarized, based on location and frequency.

Table 4. Frequency of oral self-inflicted lesions according to location.

Location of Lesion	Number	Frequency
Upper lip	6	19.36%
Lower lip	4	12.90%
Tongue	1	3.23%
Buccal mucosa	9	29.03%
Commissures	11	35.48%

Most lesions were observed at the level of oral commissures (35.48%), followed by buccal mucosa (29.03%) and the upper lip (19.36%). The lowest value was obtained for the frequency of tongue lesions (3.23%). Suggestive clinical and histopathological aspects are presented in Figures 2 and 3a,b.

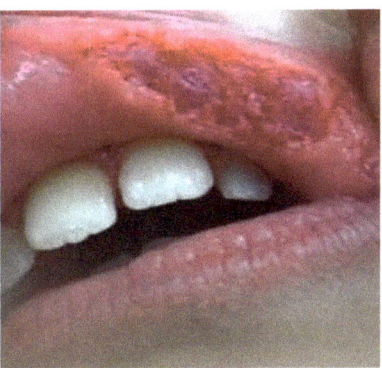

Figure 2. 14-year-old female patient, with a large wound on her upper lip, non-bleeding area of 1 × 2 cm on the non-keratinized mucosa, surrounded by erythema that did not involve the vermilion border.

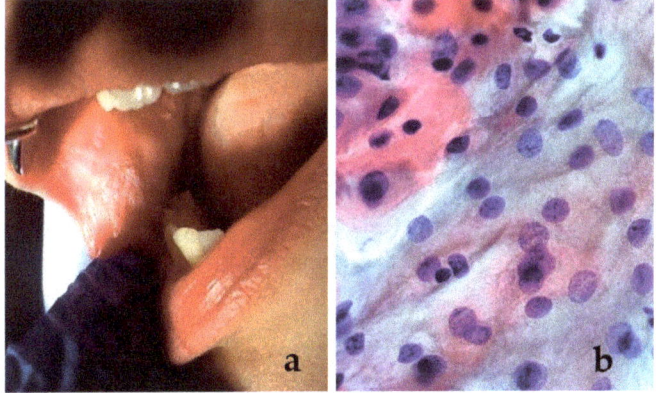

Figure 3. (**a**) A 12-year-old female patient with a white "patch" on the buccal mucosa, resembling leukoplakia; histopathological examination was performed in order to obtain the correct diagnosis; (**b**) exfoliative cytology did not confirm the presence of a premalignant lesion. Intermediate squamous cells (reflecting the accelerate turnover) with slight inflammation (different shape of nuclei, stainability, irregular contour of the nuclear border) (Papanicolaou stain, ×40).

4. Discussion

In Romania there is a large number of institutionalized children and a lack of scientific information regarding the consequences of this policy on oral health. Moreover, central Romania is multicultural and different minorities among which Hungarians and local Roma population are the most numerous. This allows a better assessment of more variables, in the effort to find possible risk factors for the development of OSH. The last few decades have been marked by increased scientific information on self-harm behavior, which could be the result of the interest of specialists or better diagnostic methods. Although considered pathological, it was reported that a large number of individuals have experienced a self-harm behavior at least once or even for a period of time in their life [18,19]. To be considered self-injury, a lesion must have the following characteristics: repetitive, socially unacceptable and to cause mild/moderate tissue damage [20]. Therefore, these lesions are usually hidden, the exact prevalence in the world is unknown and is believed to be underestimated [21]. Recent studies reported different percentages depending on the group of population analyzed, ranging from 4% in adults, 17–38% in students, 7.7–22.8% in institutionalized patients with mental disorders to 69% in high-risk young people (victims of sexual abuse or drug users) [22–25]. NSSI is a relatively common and insidious pervasive, often concealed habit that may start in childhood and increase in adolescence and young adulthood. Adolescent girls seem more vulnerable and the key components of NSSI behavior are represented by negative emotion and saturnine self-derogation [26,27].

According to data from literature, ethnicity might have an influence on self-harm behavior [28]. This was confirmed by the results of our study, as the group of local Roma showed statistically significant higher odds of developing OSH lesions compared to Romanians. The influence of ethnicity upon self-injury behavior was further confirmed by Toth et al. [29] who found that Roma population from Hungary is characterized by higher odds of developing suicidal behavior compared to non-Roma ethnics. The authors mention that studies from the UK and Hungary partially explain these tendencies by the high incidence of anxiety, depression and hostility from the majority population. For the Roma population in particular, the family concept has an important social value and, therefore, the lack of cohesion with relatives experienced by institutionalized children could be a strong negative factor for the development of anxiety and depression. These problems aggravate during adolescence and adulthood as a result of poverty, low educational level, and unemployment.

In a meta-analysis, published by Lang and Yao in 2018 [30], the estimated prevalence of NSSI in Chinese middle-school students was 22.37%, considered relatively high, females being more susceptible to this behavior (21.9% compared to a prevalence of 20.6% reported in male students). The results of our study are in accordance with this data, as out of the OSH overall prevalence of 18.1%, 13.79% were attributed to female participants and only 4.31% to male participants.

OSH is not a frequently encountered phenomenon in the daily clinical practice, but it can represent the first manifestation of a psychiatric disorder. AlSadhan et al. [31] found a higher prevalence of OSH among institutionalized children from Saudi Arabia, including gingival or mucosal lesions, cheek and lip biting. Traumatic lesions of the lips, accompanied by loss of tissue were recognized by many authors as the most frequent injuries of the oral mucosa. [32] This was explained by the proximity of incisors and canines, teeth with sharp cusps and incisal margins. In our study, the distribution of injuries is in accordance with scientific data, as the oral commissure and lips were affected in 35.48% and 32.26% cases, respectively, while the tongue was injured only in 3.23% cases. The frequent lesion of the oral commissure could be explained by the presence of caliculus angularis, a small projection of keratinized mucosa, easily injured between upper and lower canine, associated with a decreased level of pain.

Based on the literature, children who self-harm claim to have little to no pain while they are hurting themselves but they feel tension and anger towards themselves or others. This was observed also by our investigators, as none of the children who presented with OSH complained about pain during examination. A drawback of our study is that during the oral examination no psychological assessment was performed and, therefore, the tension or anger could not be quantified. It is estimated that the incidence of habitual self-injurers is nearly 1% of the population with a higher proportion of females than males, the typical onset of self-harming acts is usually at puberty. This behavior lasts 5–10 years but it can persist much longer without the proper treatment [33,34]. Institutionalized children show an increased prevalence of oral habits and OSH, which indicate emotional stress. Moreover, foster caregivers frequently lack information on these subjects and are unable to provide the proper support for these children [31].

In a study from 2015, Tortorici et al. [35] reported that oral soft tissue injuries had an incidence estimated at 2.5% in the Caucasian population. In our study group, a chronic evolution was suspected in 6 cases with OSH (5.17%) and these were further investigated using exfoliative cytology, the results confirming the benign evolution, with mild inflammation. The bite of the lips and buccal mucosa can destroy the superficial epithelium and if this parafunction has a chronic evolution, it can cause keratinized shreds or erosive and desquamative areas. These lesions can be easily identified by clinical inspection and are often related to psychologically tense persons [36]. However, in some cases, the lesions were mistaken for serious medical conditions and biopsies were required in order to rule out a malignancy. Therefore, it is important to perform a thorough clinical examination and to interpret the laboratory tests clearly [37].

4.1. Clinical Relevance

Identification of NSSI in the early stages is of utmost importance as scientific data confirm that up to 70% of these persons experienced also suicidal attempts [33]. Data from literature suggests that early age at which children engage in NSSI represents a risk factor for more episodes of NSSI during the lifetime with increased severity [17]. As self-injuries are conducted mainly in secret and may not be clearly visible, the periodic oral examination of these children might be useful in early diagnosis. Although minor OSH does not lead to a serious loss of tissue, it may affect oral health in the long run, with important social and emotional implications. Our results raise the question regarding efficient preventive measures, such as better training of caregivers and policies focusing on the psychosocial well-being of institutionalized children. Measures aiming to enhance subjective happiness and satisfaction with life at any age might decrease the prevalence of NSSI among institutionalized children [17].

4.2. Strengths and Limitations

According to our knowledge there were no studies addressing self-harm behavior of oral soft tissues in children from central Romania. However, our study encountered several limitations: the small sample size and cross-sectional design, which allowed a rapid and cost-effective evaluation of the prevalence of OSH, but is unable to provide a clear association between investigated variables. Therefore, longitudinal studies on the general population are required for a better understanding of these emotional disorders. Moreover, cognitive assessment of these children would have been useful in order to adjust confounding factors.

Author Contributions: Conceptualization, A.M.S. and M.M.; methodology, O.E.S.; software, A.M.P.; validation, A.M.S. and M.M.; formal analysis, M.M.; investigation, O.E.S. and R.E.V.; data curation, O.E.S. and R.E.V.; writing—original draft preparation, A.M.S., O.E.S., R.E.V. and A.M.P.; writing—review and editing, M.M.; supervision, A.M.P. and M.M. All authors have read and agreed to the published version of the manuscript.

Funding: This research received no external funding.

Institutional Review Board Statement: The study was conducted according to the guidelines of the Declaration of Helsinki, and approved by the Ethics Committee of the George Emil Palade University of Medicine, Pharmacy, Science, and Technology of Târgu Mureș (protocol code 520/21.11.2019).

Informed Consent Statement: Informed consent was obtained from all subjects involved in the study.

Data Availability Statement: The data presented in this study are available on request from the corresponding author. The data are not publicly available due to privacy restrictions.

Conflicts of Interest: The authors declare no conflict of interest.

References

1. Klonsky, E.D.; Muehlenkamp, J.J. Self-injury: A research review for the practitioner. *J. Clin. Psychol.* **2007**, *63*, 1045–1056. [CrossRef] [PubMed]
2. Walsh, B. Clinical assessment of self-injury: A practical guide. *J. Clin. Psychol.* **2007**, *63*, 1057–1068. [CrossRef]
3. Greydanus, D.E.; Shek, D. Deliberate self-harm and suicide in adolescents. *Keio J. Med.* **2009**, *58*, 144–151. [CrossRef]
4. Skegg, K. Self-harm. *Lancet* **2005**, *366*, 1471–1483. [CrossRef]
5. Rosenthal, E. A Mandate to End Placement of Children in Institutions and Orphanages: The Duty of Governments and Donors to Prevent Segregation and Torture (16 February 2017). *Prot. Child. Torture Deten. Glob. Solut. Glob. Probl.* **2017**. Available online: https://ssrn.com/abstract=3271306 (accessed on 12 November 2020).
6. Dozier, M.; Zeanah, C.H.; Wallin, A.R.; Shauffer, C. Institutional Care for Young Children: Review of Literature and Policy Implications. *Soc. Issues Policy Rev.* **2012**, *6*, 1–25. [CrossRef]
7. Nsabimana, E.; Rutembesa, E.; Wilhelm, P.; Martin-Soelch, C. Effects of Institutionalization and Parental Living Status on Children's Self-Esteem, and Externalizing and Internalizing Problems in Rwanda. *Front. Psychiatry* **2019**, *10*, 442. [CrossRef]
8. Vajani, M.; Annest, J.L.; Crosby, A.E.; Alexander, J.D.; Millet, L.M. Nonfatal and fatal self-harm injuries among children aged 10–14 years—United States and Oregon, 2001–2003. *Suicide Life Threat. Behav.* **2007**, *37*, 493–506. [CrossRef]
9. Limeres, J.; Feijoo, J.F.; Baluja, F.; Seoane, J.M.; Diniz, M.; Diz, P. Oral self-injury: An update. *Dent. Traumatol.* **2013**, *29*, 8–14. [CrossRef]
10. Johnson, D.E.; Tang, A.; Almas, A.N.; Degnan, K.A.; McLaughlin, K.A.; Nelson, C.A.; Fox, N.A.; CZeanah, C.H.; Drury, S.S. Caregiving Disruptions Affect Growth and Pubertal Development in Early Adolescence in Institutionalized and Fostered Romanian Children: A Randomized Clinical Trial. *J. Pediatr.* **2018**, *203*, 345–353.e3. [CrossRef]
11. Sonuga-Barke, E.J.S.; Kennedy, M.; Kumsta, R.; Knights, N.; Golm, D.; Rutter, M.; Maughan, B.; Schlotz, W.; Kreppner, J. Child-to-adult neurodevelopmental and mental health trajectories after early life deprivation: The young adult follow-up of the longitudinal English and Romanian Adoptees study. *Lancet* **2017**, *389*, 1539–1548. [CrossRef]
12. Dobrova-Krol, N.A.; van Ijzendoorn, M.H.; Bakermans-Kranenburg, M.J.; Cyr, C.; Juffer, F. Physical growth delays and stress dysregulation in stunted and non-stunted Ukrainian institution-reared children. *Infant Behav. Dev.* **2008**, *31*, 539–553. [CrossRef] [PubMed]
13. Warner, H.A.; McCall, R.B.; Groark, C.J.; Kim, K.H.; Muhamedrahimov, R.J.; Palmov, O.I.; Nikiforova, N.V. Caregiver-child interaction, caregiver transitions, and group size as mediators between intervention condition and attachment and physical growth outcomes in institutionalized children. *Infant Ment. Health J.* **2017**, *38*, 645–657. [CrossRef] [PubMed]
14. Flemming, M.; Aronson, L. Child Maltreatment and Non-Suicidal Self-Injury. Information Brief Series, Cornell Research Program on Self-Injury and Recovery. Cornell University Ithaca, NY. 2016. Available online: http://www.selfinjury.bctr.cornell.edu/perch/resources/the-relationship-between-child-maltreatment-and-non-suicidal-self-injuryfinal.pdf (accessed on 20 August 2020).
15. DiPierro, R.; Samo, I.; Perego, S.; Galucci, M.; Madeddu, F. Adolescent non-suicidal self-injury: The effects of personality traits, family relationship and maltreatment on the presence and severity of behaviours. *Eur. Child Adolesc. Psychiatry* **2012**, *21*, 511–520. [CrossRef]
16. Lang, C.M.; Sharma-Patel, K. The relation between childhood maltreatment and self-injury: A review of the literature on conceptualization and intervention. *Trauma Violence Abuse* **2011**, *12*, 23–37. [CrossRef]
17. Muehlenkamp, J.J.; Xhunga, N.; Brausch, A.M. Self-injury Age of Onset: A Risk Factor for NSSI Severity and Suicidal Behavior. *Arch. Suicide Res.* **2019**, *23*, 551–563. [CrossRef]
18. Buresova, I. Self-Harm classification system development: Theoretical study. *Rev. Soc. Sci.* **2016**, *1*, 3–20. [CrossRef]

19. Madge, N.; Hewitt, A.; Hawton, K.; De Wilde, E.J.; Corcoran, P.; Fekete, S.; van Heeringan, K.; DeLeo, D.; Ystgaard, M. Deliberate self-harm within an international community sample of young people: Comparative findings from the Child & Adolescent Self-harm in Europe (CASE) Study. *J. Child Psychol. Psychiatry* **2008**, *49*, 667–677. [CrossRef]
20. Cannavale, R.; Itro, A.; Campisi, G.; Compilato, D.; Collella, G. Oral self-injuries: Clinical findings in a series of 19 patients. *Med. Oral Pathol. Oral Cir. Bucal* **2015**, *20*, e123. [CrossRef]
21. Klonsky, E.D. Non-suicidal self-injury in United States adults: Prevalence, sociodemographics, topography and functions. *Psychol. Med.* **2011**, *41*, 1981–1986. [CrossRef]
22. Gratz, K.L.; Conrad, S.D.; Roemer, L. Risk factors for deliberate self-harm among college students. *Am. J. Orthopsychiatry* **2002**, *72*, 128–140. [CrossRef]
23. Withlock, J.; Eckenrode, J.; Silverman, D. Self-injurious behaviors in a college population. *Pediatrics* **2006**, *117*, 1939–1948. [CrossRef]
24. Lloyd-Richardson, E.E.; Perrine, N.; Dierker, L.; Kelley, M.L. Characteristics and functions of non-suicidal self-injury in a community sample of adolescents. *Psychol. Med.* **2007**, *37*, 1183–1192. [CrossRef] [PubMed]
25. Wilkinson, B. Current trends in remediating adolescent self-injury: An integrative review. *J. Sch. Nurs.* **2011**, *27*, 120–128. [CrossRef] [PubMed]
26. Yates, T.M.; Carlson, E.A.; Egeland, B. A prospective study of child maltreatment and self-injurious behavior in a community sample. *Dev. Psychopathol.* **2008**, *20*, 651–671. [CrossRef] [PubMed]
27. Brunner, R.; Parzer, P.; Haffner, J. Prevalence and psychological correlates of occasional and deliberate self-harm in adolescents. *Arch. Pediatr. Adolesc. Med.* **2007**, *161*, 641–649. [CrossRef] [PubMed]
28. Portzky, G.; De Wilde, E.J.; van Heeringen, K. Deliberate self-harm in young people: Differences in prevalence and risk factors between the Netherlands and Belgium. *Eur. Child Adolesc. Psychiatry* **2008**, *17*, 179–186. [CrossRef]
29. Tóth, M.D.; Ádám, S.; Zonda, T.; Birkás, E.; Purebl, G. Risk factors for multiple suicide attempts among Roma in Hungary. *Transcult. Psychiatry* **2018**, *55*, 55–72. [CrossRef]
30. Lang, J.; Yao, Y. Prevalence of nonsuicidal self-injury in Chinese middle school and high school students. A meta-analysis. *Medicine* **2018**, *97*, e12916. [CrossRef]
31. AlSadhan, S.A.; Al-Jobair, A.M. Oral habits, dental trauma, and occlusal characteristics among 4- to 12-year-old institutionalized orphan children in Riyadh, Saudi Arabia. *Spec. Care Dent.* **2017**, *37*, 10–18. [CrossRef]
32. Millogo, M.; Ouedraogo, R.W.L.; Ily, V.; Konsem, T.; Ouedraogo, D. Labial lesions by human bite. *J. Oral Med. Oral Surg.* **2018**, *24*, 153–156. [CrossRef]
33. Kostic, J.; Zikic, O.; Stankovic, M.; Nikolic, G. Nonsuicidal self-injury among adolescents in south-east Serbia. *Int. J. Pediatr. Adolesc. Med.* **2019**, *6*, 131–134. [CrossRef] [PubMed]
34. Tang, J.; Yang, W.; Ahmed, N.I.; Ma, Y.; Liu, H.Y.; Wang, J.J.; Wang, P.X.; Du, Y.K.; Yu, Y.Z. Stressful Life Events as a Predictor for Nonsuicidal Self-Injury in Southern Chinese Adolescence. A Cross-Sectional Study. *Medicine* **2016**, *95*, e2637. [CrossRef]
35. Tortorici, S.; Corrao, S.; Natoli, G.; Difalco, P. Prevalence and distribution of oral mucosal non-malignant lesions in the western Sicilian population. *Minerva Stomatol.* **2016**, *65*, 191–206. [PubMed]
36. Hailegiorgis, M.T.; Berheto, T.M.; Sibamo, E.L.; Asseffa, N.A.; Tesfa, G.; Birhanu, F. Psychological wellbeing of children at public primary schools in Jimma town: An orphan and non-orphan comparative study. *PLoS ONE* **2018**, *13*, e0195377. [CrossRef]
37. Monea, M.; Olah, P.; Comaneanu, R.M.; Hancu, V.; Ormenisan, A. The Role of Toluidine Blue as a Visual Diagnostic Method in Oral Premalignant Lesions. *Rev. Chim.* **2016**, *67*, 1370–1372.

Publisher's Note: MDPI stays neutral with regard to jurisdictional claims in published maps and institutional affiliations.

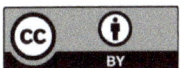

© 2020 by the authors. Licensee MDPI, Basel, Switzerland. This article is an open access article distributed under the terms and conditions of the Creative Commons Attribution (CC BY) license (http://creativecommons.org/licenses/by/4.0/).

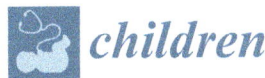

Article

Does Sex Dimorphism Exist in Dysfunctional Movement Patterns during the Sensitive Period of Adolescence?

Josip Karuc [1,*], Mario Jelčić [2], Maroje Sorić [1], Marjeta Mišigoj-Duraković [1] and Goran Marković [1,2]

[1] Faculty of Kinesiology, University of Zagreb, Horvaćanski zavoj 15, 10000 Zagreb, Croatia; maroje.soric@kif.unizg.hr (M.S.); marjeta.misigoj-durakovic@kif.unizg.hr (M.M.-D.); goran.markovic@kif.unizg.hr (G.M.)
[2] Motus Melior, Sport and Rehabilitation Center, Hektorovićeva ulica 2, 10000 Zagreb, Croatia; mjelcic1@gmail.com
* Correspondence: josip.karuc@kif.unizg.hr

Received: 26 November 2020; Accepted: 17 December 2020; Published: 20 December 2020

Abstract: This study aimed to investigate sex difference in the functional movement in the adolescent period. Seven hundred and thirty adolescents (365 boys) aged 16–17 years participated in the study. The participants performed standardized Functional Movement Screen™ (FMS^{TM}) protocol and a t-test was used to examine sex differences in the total functional movement screen score, while the chi-square test was used to determine sex differences in the proportion of dysfunctional movement and movement asymmetries within the individual FMS^{TM} tests. Girls demonstrated higher total FMS^{TM} score compared to boys (12.7 ± 2.3 and 12.2 ± 2.4, respectively; $p = 0.0054$). Sex differences were present in several individual functional movement patterns where boys demonstrated higher prevalence of dysfunctional movement compared to girls in patterns that challenge mobility and flexibility of the body (inline lunge: 32% vs. 22%, $df = 1$, $p = 0.0009$; shoulder mobility: 47% vs. 26%, $df = 1$, $p < 0.0001$; and active straight leg raise: 31% vs. 9%, $df = 1$, $p < 0.0001$), while girls underperformed in tests that have higher demands for upper-body strength and abdominal stabilization (trunk stability push-up: 81% vs. 44%, $df = 1$, $p < 0.0001$; and rotary stability: 54% vs. 44%, $df = 1$, $p = 0.0075$). Findings of this study suggest that sex dimorphisms exist in functional movement patterns in the period of mid-adolescence. The results of this research need to be considered while using FMS^{TM} as a screening tool, as well as the reference standard for exercise intervention among the secondary school-aged population.

Keywords: FMS^{TM}; pubescence; maturation; fundamental movement patterns; functional movement; gender difference

1. Introduction

Physical inactivity represents a global health problem and is related to higher risk for morbidity and mortality [1]. Evidence has shown that inactive children are exposed to increased cardiometabolic risk [2,3]. Physical activity in childhood and adolescence is important to attain appropriate bone mineral content [4]. Although the influence of physical activity as a measure of movement quantity has been examined extensively, very few studies have examined the movement quality through the sensitive period of adolescence. However, these studies pointed out the importance of proper development of the optimal functional movement patterns through adolescence [5–16]. Since functional movement is considered the clinical measure of movement quality [17,18] and potentially the essential component for optimal motor development, the investigation of the optimal functional movement in childhood and adolescence needs special attention.

Functional movement can be defined as optimal flexibility of the soft tissue, mobility of the joints, and neuromuscular control of the body regions involved in the particular motor task [17,18]. On the other hand, dysfunctional movement (DFM) is characterized by movement compensations evident across the kinematic chain with a significant loss in mobility, observed asymmetry, and poor movement control of the particular motor task [17,18]. The importance of functional movement patterns has been studied widely [19–21] and they represent the basic foundation for the execution of more complex motor tasks [17,18]. A higher incidence of musculoskeletal injury has been associated with DFM patterns among the athletic population [19–21], while some studies reported the opposite [22–24]. The most common diagnostic tool to assess functional movement is Functional Movement Screen (FMS^{TM}) which evaluates mobility and stability in seven functional movement patterns: deep squat, hurdle step, inline lunge, shoulder mobility, active straight leg raise (ASLR), trunk stability push-up, and rotary stability [17,18]. FMS^{TM} can detect movement asymmetries if a difference between the right and left side of the uni/contralateral movement patterns is observed [17,18]. What is more, the literature shows that movement asymmetries detected via FMS^{TM} have been associated with higher injury risk [5] which could possibly contribute to the development of musculoskeletal deformities in later life.

The presence of the DFM patterns and movement asymmetries in childhood could facilitate postural abnormalities in the period of mid-adolescence. Indeed, evidence shows that neuromuscular control of the movement is not properly developed by the time of the adolescent period [25]. Therefore, identifying DFM patterns and movement asymmetries in this period of a child's growth needs special attention. Still, only a few studies have investigated sex differences in functional movement in an average or athletic adolescent population. These studies suggest that, in both the general and athletic population, girls exhibit better functional movement compared to boys [8–10,12,15,16], while some studies reported opposite or no difference between sexes [6,11,13,14]. However, these were either small-scale studies [11–13] or included only active adolescents [5–10,14] or adolescents with overweight/obesity [7] and did not analyze movement asymmetries.

However, to this date, none of the studies have investigated sex differences in functional movement and movement asymmetries in a large representative sample of school-aged mid-adolescents. Therefore, the purpose of this study was to examine sex dimorphism in functional movement patterns and movement asymmetries in the representative sample of mid-adolescents.

2. Materials and Methods

2.1. Participants

This investigation is a part of the Croatian physical activity in adolescence longitudinal study (CRO-PALS) conducted in a representative sample of urban youth (city of Zagreb, Croatia). This study was performed during the second wave of assessments, and all measurements were taken in 2015, during March, April, and May. Information about the procedures of the CRO-PALS longitudinal study have been documented in previous research [26]. In brief, using stratified two-stage random sampling procedures (school level and class level), 54 classes in 14 secondary schools were selected to participate in the CRO-PALS study (schools were stratified by type: grammar schools/vocational schools/private schools). All 1408 students in the selected classes were approached, and 903 agreed to participate (response rate = 64%). One hundred and twenty participants were unavailable on the day of testing or did not complete the FMS^{TM} screening. Of one hundred and twenty participants, one hundred and seventeen were unavailable on the day of testing because they were missing from the school at the time of the measurements, whereas three subjects did not complete FMS^{TM} screening due to lack of time (1 girl and 2 boys). As a consequence, we included data from 783 adolescents. All the participants had to meet certain criteria for the medical doctor to perform the screening process, specifically: (1) not having any pain during the movement screening (i.e., FMS^{TM} testing procedures), (2) not having an acute medical condition that precluded FMS^{TM} testing (neurologic disorders or serious orthopedic trauma such as bone fractures or complete muscle ruptures). Accordingly, 53 subjects were excluded. Therefore, the total number of participants that were analyzed was 730 (girls, n = 368, mean age ± SD = 16.6 ± 0.4 years old (yo), mean weight ± SD = 60.1 ± 9.3, mean height ± SD = 166.3 ± 6.4; boys, n = 362, mean age ± SD = 16.7 ± 0.4 yo, mean weight ± SD = 71.7 ± 12.5, mean height ± SD = 179.0 ± 7.2). The flowchart of the included participants is shown in Figure 1.

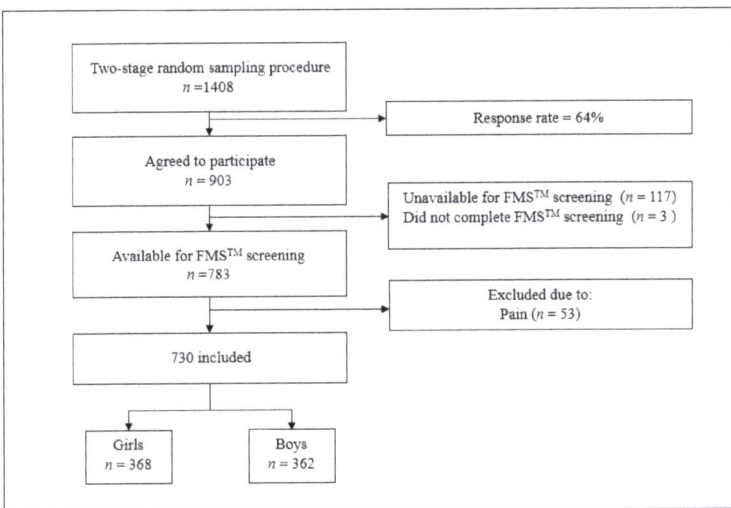

Figure 1. Flowchart of included participants.

Children and their parents were fully informed about the purposes of the research, its protocols, and possible hazards and discomforts related to the procedures used. Written consent was obtained from both children and their parents or legal guardians. The study was performed according to the Declaration of Helsinki and the procedures were approved by the Ethics Committee of the Faculty of Kinesiology, University of Zagreb (No: 1009-2014).

2.2. Functional Movement Screen

FMS^{TM} is an instrument designed for the evaluation of mobility and stability of seven functional movement tests: the deep squat, hurdle step, inline lunge, shoulder mobility, ASLR, trunk stability push-up, and rotary stability [17,18]. In the current study, ten novice trained raters used FMS^{TM} according to the official guidelines. All ten raters passed a two-day FMS^{TM} education course by an FMS^{TM} certified practitioner. Despite a large number of raters recruited in this study, previous research reported moderate to good interrater and intra-rater reliability of the FMS^{TM} among novice raters [27,28]. Participants had a maximum of three trials for each test in accordance with the recommended protocol [17,18] while each test was scored on a four-point scale, from 0 to 3, with higher scores indicating better functional movement. Evidence shows that pain can alter movement control [29]. Therefore, subjects were asked if they felt pain during the FMS^{TM} assessment and were subsequently scored with a score of 0 and excluded if they answered this question positively (n = 53). In the current study, a functional movement was defined as the movement with a given score of 2 or 3 during FMS^{TM} testing. Also, a score of 1 was recorded when the participant was unable to perform the movement task due to the number of movement compensations present, which reflects the DFM pattern [17,18]. This means that a score of 2 and 3 was an indicator of functional movement, whereas a score of 1 was an indicator of DFM for each of the 7 individual FMS^{TM} tests. If a discrepancy in the scores between the right and left side of the contra/unilateral FMS^{TM} test was observed, movement asymmetry was documented for that specific FMS^{TM} test. We analyzed movement asymmetries for five contra/unilateral FMS^{TM} tests (i.e., hurdle step, inline lunge, shoulder mobility, ASLR, and rotary stability). Accordingly, number (n) and proportion (%) of subjects who performed DFM or showed movement asymmetry could be calculated in each of the seven or five individual FMS^{TM} movement patterns, respectively. This was the basic step for analyzing the differences in the proportion of participants who performed DFM or demonstrated any asymmetry between girls and boys for individual FMS^{TM} tests (i.e., using chi-square tests). In addition, the total FMS^{TM} score was set as an outcome continuous variable and was calculated according to the literature [17,18].

2.3. Sport Participation

In order to assess whether someone participated in an organized sport activity or not, the questionnaire was offered with two YES/NO questions inquiring about regular participation in organized sports in school, as well as outside of the school. For participants who stated that they participated in organized sport, a comprehensive list of sports activities was offered and participants identified all the sports in which they regularly participated.

2.4. Statistical Analysis

An independent *t*-test was used to examine differences between sexes in total FMS^{TM} score. Chi-square test was performed to investigate differences between girls and boys in the proportion of DFM in 7 individual FMS^{TM} tests and for the movement asymmetries exhibited in the 5 contralateral FMS^{TM} tests. In addition, the same analyses concerning sex differences were done for the group of non-athletic and athletic participants separately. Data are presented as mean ± SD. All analyses were performed using Statistica (version 13.0) and the level of statistical significance was set at $p < 0.05$.

3. Results

The basic characteristics of participants are shown in Table 1. Results demonstrated that girls slightly outperformed boys in total FMS^{TM} score (12.7 ± 2.4 and 12.2 ± 25, respectively; $p = 0.0054$).

Table 1. Basic characteristics of participants by sex.

Basic Characteristics		Girls	Boys
BMI (kg/m^2) Mean (SD)		21.7 (3.2)	22.4 (3.5)
Waist Circumference (cm) Mean (SD)		68.7 (6.4)	76.0 (7.5)
Hips Circumference (cm) Mean (SD)		96.7 (7.5)	98.0 (7.5)
Sum of Four Skinfolds (mm) Mean (SD)		48.8 (15.0)	37.1 (18.1)
Functional Movement Asymmetries n (%)	0	76 (21)	86 (23)
	1	128 (35)	126 (34)
	2	98 (27)	111 (30)
	3	51 (14)	38 (10)
	4	7 (2)	7 (2)
	5	2 (0.5)	0 (0)
Sport Participation * n (%)		93 (25)	173 (48)
SES Median (IQR)		3 (1)	2 (1)

Note: BMI: Body Mass Index; Functional Movement Asymmetries n (%): Number (n) and percentage (%) of participants who exhibited Functional Movement Asymmetries within each sex group; Sport Participation n (%): Number (n) and percentage (%) of participants that participated in sport activity; SES: Socioeconomic status (1—Much lower than average, 2—Lower than average, 3—Average, 4—Higher than average, 5—Much higher than average); IQR: Interquartile Range; SD: Standard Deviation; * Data are presented for 725 participants.

Figure 2 depicts the proportion (%) of DFM patterns among girls and boys in all seven FMS^{TM} tests. Girls demonstrated a higher proportion of DFM patterns compared to boys in trunk stability push-up (81% vs. 44%, $df = 1$, $p < 0.0001$) and rotary stability (54% vs. 44%, $df = 1$, $p = 0.0075$). However, boys showed a higher proportion of DFM in inline lunge (32% vs. 22%, $df = 1$, $p = 0.0009$), shoulder mobility (47% vs. 26%, $df = 1$, $p < 0.0001$), and ASLR (31% vs. 9%, $df = 1$, $p < 0.0001$), while scores in deep squat and hurdle step were similar in both sexes (see Figure 2).

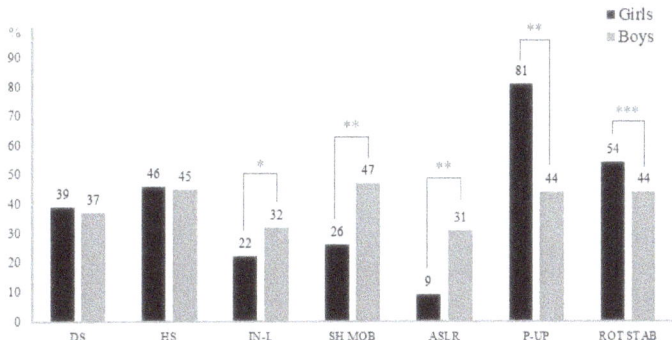

Figure 2. Proportion (%) of adolescent girls and boys who performed dysfunctional movement (DFM) in each Functional Movement Screen™ (FMS™) test. Note: DS: deep squat; HS: hurdle step; IN-L: inline lunge; SHO MOB: shoulder mobility; ASLR: active straight leg raise; P-UP: Trunk stability push-up; ROT STAB: rotary stability. * $p = 0.0009$; ** $p < 0.0001$; *** $p = 0.0075$.

Boys demonstrated a higher proportion of movement asymmetries compared to girls in shoulder mobility (45% vs. 36%, $df = 1$, $p = 0.0218$) and ASLR (21% vs. 13%, $df = 1$, $p = 0.008$). However, no significant difference between girls and boys in the proportion of the movement asymmetries was found for the other FMS™ tests: hurdle step (27% vs. 24%, $df = 1$, $p = 0.331$), inline lunge (31% vs. 31%, $df = 1$, $p = 0.95$), and rotary stability (26% vs. 22%, $df = 1$, $p = 0.237$) (see Figure 3).

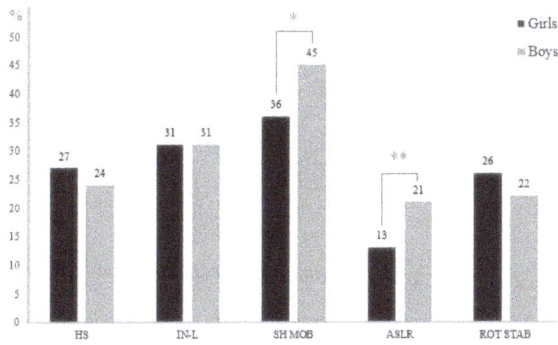

Figure 3. Proportion (%) of adolescent girls and boys who demonstrated movement asymmetries in each FMS™ test. Note: HS: hurdle step; IN-L: inline lunge; SHO MOB: shoulder mobility; ASLR: active straight leg raise; ROT STAB: rotary stability. * $p = 0.0218$; ** $p = 0.008$.

Subgroup Analyses

Since five subjects did not report sport participation status (due to being absent from school), all subgroup analyses were based on 725 participants. When the sample was stratified by sport participation, within the group of non-athletic participants there was no sex differences in the total FMS^{TM} score (girls vs. boys, 12.6 vs. 12.2, respectively, $p = 0.11$). However, among the athletic subgroup of adolescents, girls significantly outperformed boys (13.2 vs. 12.3, $p = 0.002$). Among the non-athletic adolescents, boys demonstrated higher proportion of DFM in three tests compared to girls (inline lunge: 24% vs. 33%, $df = 1$, $p = 0.032$; shoulder mobility: 29% vs. 41%, $df = 1$, $p = 0.004$; ASLR: 7% vs. 34%, $df = 1$, $p < 0.0001$). On the other hand, girls underperformed in push-up and rotary stability tests (push up: 80% vs. 44%, $df = 1$; $p < 0.0001$; rotary stability: 56% vs. 47%, $df = 1$; $p = 0.04$), while in squat and hurdle step patterns no sex differences were shown ($p = 0.25$–0.66). In addition, non-athletic boys showed a lesser number of asymmetries compared to non-athletic girls in the shoulder mobility test (50% vs. 67%, $df = 1$, $p = 0.01$), while other four uni/contralateral tests failed to reach significance ($p = 0.06$–0.4).

Among the subgroup of adolescents who have participated in sports, girls showed a lesser proportion of DFM compared to boys in inline lunge (13% vs. 31%, $df = 1$; $p = 0.0009$), shoulder mobility (20% vs. 51%, $df = 1$, $p < 0.0001$), and ASLR (11% vs. 28%, $df = 1$, $p = 0.001$). On the other hand, boys exhibited a lesser proportion of the DFM in the push-up test (43% vs. 85%, $df = 1$, $p < 0.0001$). However, there was no significant sex difference observed in squat, hurdle step, and rotary stability ($p = 0.41$–0.61). Concerning movement asymmetries, athletic girls demonstrated a lesser proportion of the asymmetries only in the ASLR movement pattern (13% vs. 22%, $df = 1$, $p = 0.018$).

4. Discussion

This study aimed to determine functional movement status in a general adolescent population. The main finding of this study is that adolescent boys showed a higher proportion of DFM and movement asymmetries in the larger number of FMS^{TM} tests compared to adolescent girls. More specifically, boys demonstrated a higher proportion of DFM and movement asymmetries in the inline lunge, shoulder mobility, and ASLR tests, which could potentially predispose them to higher injury for lower and upper extremities [5]. On the other hand, girls demonstrated a higher prevalence of DFM in the push-up and rotary stability tests. A low score in the trunk stability pushup test and rotary stability could indicate inadequate reactive stabilization of the trunk muscles and a deficit in the upper body strength in the female adolescent population [18]. For this reason, adolescent girls in the current study could be more prone to suffer from a higher risk of lower back injury [30]. On the other hand, girls slightly outperformed boys in total FMS^{TM} score (12.7 vs. 12.3 points) which further emphasized the aforementioned sex difference in functional movement during the mid-adolescent period.

In the current study, when the sample was stratified by sport participation, subgroup analyses showed similar results when compared to the findings of the initial analysis (i.e., for the total sample). The main difference between findings from the total sample and subsample was in the total FMS^{TM} score. More specifically, athletic girls outperformed athletic boys significantly (13.2 vs. 12.3, respectively), whereas in the subgroup of non-athletic participants sex difference was not noted. However, when the proportion of DFM and asymmetries are considered, similar patterns of movement dysfunction can be seen in both the athletic and non-athletic subgroup of participants, as well as within the total sample of mid-adolescents. This could possibly mean that sport participation probably does not influence functional movement status in the adolescent period since similar patterns of movement dysfunction were observed within the aforementioned groups and subgroups of mid-adolescents. Indeed, according to the current literature, in both the general and athletic adolescent population, most evidence demonstrates that females have a higher total FMS^{TM} score compared to males [8–10,12,15,16], although two studies reported opposite results [6,14]. In the study done by Abraham et al. [14], a large age span (10–17 yo) among participants revealed that pre-pubertal and pubertal subjects were included in the sample and all inactive children were excluded, which could potentially lead to higher mean values. Some researchers found no sex difference in total FMS^{TM} score [11,13], which could be potentially contributed to different populations studied (8-11 yo) and much smaller sample sizes (n = 77 and n = 58, respectively). Concerning individual FMS^{TM} patterns, evidence almost consistently shows that, in both general and athletic adolescents, same sex differences are present. More specifically, female adolescents generally show a better quality of movement in flexibility/mobility tests [10,11,13,16] while boys are better at push up and rotary stability [6,11,13–16]. Reported results from previous studies are in line with the findings of our study. What our study adds to the existing body of knowledge is that the same sex differences in functional movement exist in the population of mid-adolescents.

Still, it remains unanswered as to why these sex differences in the functional movement patterns are present in the adolescent period. Therefore, three possible explanations for observed phenomena should be considered. *(1) Physiological—potential effect of maturation on muscle performance*: girls scored higher in the inline lunge, shoulder mobility, and ASLR, which could be due to higher mobility/flexibility demands of these movements [17,18]. This could be further explained with previous findings that reported greater mobility among girls compared to boys during the adolescent period of growth [31]. Since higher values of upper body strength are reported in boys compared to girls during adolescence [32], this could explain the discrepancy that was found in the upper body test (i.e., trunk stability push-up). *(2) Anatomical—potential effect of sex on joint morphology*: Reported differences in the aforementioned FMS^{TM} patterns could be possibly due to different architecture of the pelvis, hip, and shoulder since adolescent girls demonstrate more general joint laxity, hip anteversion, and tibiofemoral angles compared to adolescent boys [33]. Furthermore, development of the adolescent female pelvis from fifteen years of age and onward differs considerably from males, which can contribute to observed discrepancies in reported DFM in the current study [34]. The difference in the proportion of DFM in lower body patterns reported in the current study could be due to different hip architecture since it has been shown that adolescent girls have a different orientation of the acetabulum compared to boys [35]. More specifically, girls from the age of 13 to 17 have increased acetabular anteversion compared to boys [35]. This could possibly explain why girls performed better on tasks that demand active hip flexion (i.e., inline lunge and ASLR), whereas the different orientation of the acetabulum in boys could limit hip flexion movements. What could be concerning is that a higher prevalence of DFM observed in lower body patterns among boys could predispose them to a higher risk for developing hip orthopedic abnormalities (i.e., femoroacetabular impingement) [36]. *(3) Sociocultural—potential effect of cultural engagement in specific sport activity*: adolescent boys tend to engage more in sports such as soccer and basketball which have a high prevalence of unilateral and asymmetrical movement patterns [37]. This could further facilitate movement asymmetries seen in shoulder mobility and ASLR tests. On the other hand, girls participate more in sport activities that have an aesthetic component (i.e., dance, ballet, etc.) where specific unilateral movement patterns are not emphasized or trained in isolation [37]. Given the fact that in the current study more boys were engaged in sport activity compared to girls (48% vs. 25%, respectively), the aforementioned explanations could possibly explaine behind mechanism for observed discrepancies between adolescent girls and boys concerning movement asymmetries.

This study has several strengths. First, this is the only study that provides information about dysfunctional movement as well as movement asymmetries assessed by FMS^{TM} in a large sample of urban adolescents. Second, this is the first study to investigate a highly age-homogenized adolescent population (16–17 yo). Third, current research is based on a reasonably large number of participants (n = 733). All this allowed for more precise information about sex differences in a functional movement to be investigated. However, there are also several limitations that need to be considered while interpreting this data. This study investigated a population in the urban area, thus excluding children from rural areas which may affect the generalizability of the results in the context of the whole adolescent population. The large number of raters used in this study can be a potential drawback, although good interrater agreement in FMS^{TM} scores has been repeatedly reported [27,28]. Despite all this, the results of the present study give comprehensive data about a functional movement among the adolescent population.

5. Conclusions

The results of this study confirmed some previous findings and offer a new perspective in the context of functional movement in an adolescent population. In the current study, the total functional movement screen score was higher in girls compared to boys. Sex differences were present in several individual functional movement patterns, where boys demonstrated a higher prevalence of DFM in patterns that challenged mobility and flexibility of the body, while girls underperformed in tests that had higher demands for upper body strength and abdominal stabilization. The results of the present study need to be considered while implementing data into practical usage and while using FMS^{TM} as a screening tool among an adolescent school-aged population. Future research should focus on investigating sex dimorphism in functional movement in other populations of children and adolescents.

Author Contributions: Conceptualization: J.K., M.J., M.S., M.M.-D. and G.M.; data curation: M.S. and M.M.-D.; formal analysis: J.K., M.J., M.S. and G.M.; funding acquisition: M.S. and M.M.-D.; investigation: J.K., M.J., M.S., M.M.-D. and G.M.; methodology: J.K., M.J., M.S., M.M.-D. and G.M.; project administration: M.S. and M.M.-D.; resources: M.S., M.M.-D. and G.M.; software: J.K., M.S. and G.M.; supervision: M.S., M.M.-D. and G.M.; validation, J.K., M.J., M.S., M.M.-D. and G.M.; visualization: J.K. and M.J.; writing original draft: J.K., M.J. and M.S.; writing review & editing: J.K., M.J., M.S., M.M.-D. and G.M. All authors have read and agreed to the published version of the manuscript.

Funding: This work is a part of the Croatian physical activity in adolescence longitudinal study (CRO-PALS), funded by the Croatian Science Foundation under the grant no. IP-2016-06-9926, and grant no: DOK-2018-01-2328.

Acknowledgments: The authors would like to thank L. Blaževic, M. Stepić, Pašuld S. Venier M., A. Trbojević, F. Bolčević, M. Bičanić, and R. Buljanović, for help concerning the FMS^{TM} assessment.

Conflicts of Interest: The authors declare no conflict of interest.

References

1. Warburton, D.; Charlesworth, S.; Ivey, A.; Nettlefold, L.; Bredin, S.S. A systematic review of the evidence for Canada's Physical Activity Guidelines for Adults. *Int. J. Behav. Nutr. Phys. Act.* **2010**, *7*, 39. [CrossRef] [PubMed]
2. Ekelund, U.; Anderssen, S.A.; Froberg, K.; Sardinha, L.N.; Andersen, L.B.; Brage, S. Independent associations of physical activity and cardiorespiratory fitness with metabolic risk factors in children: The European youth heart study. *Diabetologia* **2007**, *50*, 18320–18400. [CrossRef] [PubMed]
3. Andersen, L.B.; Harro, M.; Sardinha, L.B.; Froberg, K.; Ekelund, U.; Brage, S.; Anderssen, S.A. Physical activity and clustered cardiovascular risk in children: A cross-sectional study (The European Youth Heart Study). *Lancet* **2006**, *368*, 299–304. [CrossRef]
4. Ondrak, K.S.; Morgan, D.W. Physical Activity, Calcium Intake and Bone Health in Children and Adolescents. *Sports Med.* **2007**, *37*, 587–600. [CrossRef]
5. Chalmers, S.; Fuller, J.T.; De Benedictis, T.A.; Townsley, S.; Lynagh, M.; Gleeson, C.; Zacharia, A.; Thomson, S.; Magarey, M. Asymmetry during preseason Functional Movement Screen testing is associated with injury during a junior Australian football season. *J. Sci. Med. Sport* **2017**, *20*, 653–657. [CrossRef]
6. Anderson, B.E.; Neumann, M.L.; Bliven, K.C.H. Functional Movement Screen Differences Between Male and Female Secondary School Athletes. *J. Strength Cond. Res.* **2015**, *29*, 1098–1106. [CrossRef]
7. Molina-Garcia, P.; Migueles, J.H.; Cadenas-Sanchez, C.; Esteban-Cornejo, I.; Mora-Gonzalez, J.; Rodriguez-Ayllon, M.; Plaza-Florido, A.; Molina-Molina, A.; Garcia-Delgado, G.; D'Hondt, E.; et al. Fatness and fitness in relation to functional movement quality in overweight and obese children. *J. Sports Sci.* **2019**, *37*, 878–885. [CrossRef]
8. Paszkewicz, J.R.; Mccarty, C.W.; Van Lunen, B. Comparison of Functional and Static Evaluation Tools among Adolescent Athletes. *J. Strength Cond. Res.* **2013**, *27*, 2842–2850. [CrossRef]

9. Kramer, T.A.; Sacko, R.S.; Pfeifer, C.E.; Gatens, D.R.; Goins, J.M.; Stodden, D.F. The association between the Functional Movement Screen™, Y-balance test, and physical performance tests in male and female high school athletes. *Int. J. Sports Phys. Ther.* **2019**, *14*, 911–919. [CrossRef]
10. Pfeifer, C.E.; Sacko, R.S.; Ortaglia, A.; Monsma, E.V.; Beattie, P.F.; Goins, J.; Stodden, D.F. Functional movement Screen™ in youth sport participants: Evaluating the proficiency barrier for injury. *Int. J. Sports Phys. Ther.* **2019**, *14*, 436–444. [CrossRef]
11. Mitchell, U.H.; Johnson, A.W.; Adamson, B. Relationship Between Functional Movement Screen Scores, Core Strength, Posture, and Body Mass Index in School Children in Moldova. *J. Strength Cond. Res.* **2015**, *29*, 1172–1179. [CrossRef] [PubMed]
12. Duncan, M.J.; Stanley, M. Functional Movement Is Negatively Associated with Weight Status and Positively Associated with Physical Activity in British Primary School Children. *J. Obes.* **2012**, *2012*, 1–5. [CrossRef] [PubMed]
13. Duncan, M.J.; Stanley, M.; Leddington-Wright, S. The association between functional movement and overweight and obesity in British primary school children. *Sports Med. Arthrosc. Rehabil. Ther. Technol.* **2013**, *5*, 1–8. [CrossRef] [PubMed]
14. Abraham, A.; Sannasi, R.; Nair, R. Normative values for the functional movement Screen™ in adolescent school aged children. *Int. J. Sports Phys. Ther.* **2015**, *10*, 29–36. [PubMed]
15. García-Pinillos, F.; Roche-Seruendo, L.E.; Delgado-Floody, P.; Mayorga, D.J.; Latorre-Román, P.Á. Original is there any relationship between functional movement and weight status. *Nutr. Hosp.* **2018**, *35*, 805–810. [CrossRef]
16. O'Brien, W.; Duncan, M.J.; Farmer, O.; Lester, D. Do Irish Adolescents Have Adequate Functional Movement Skill and Confidence? *J. Mot. Learn. Dev.* **2018**, *6*, S301–S319. [CrossRef]
17. Cook, G.; Burton, L.; Hoogenboom, B. Pre-Participation Screening: The Use of Fundamental Movements as an Assessment of Function—Part 1. *N. Am. J. Sport. Phys. Ther.* **2006**, *1*, 62–72. [CrossRef]
18. Cook, G.; Burton, L.; Hoogenboom, B. Pre-Participation Screening: The Use of Fundamental Movements as an Assessment of Function—Part 2. *N. Am. J. Sport. Phys. Ther.* **2006**, *1*, 132–139. [CrossRef]
19. Kiesel, K.B.; Butler, R.J.; Plisky, P.J. Prediction of Injury by Limited and Asymmetrical Fundamental Movement Patterns in American Football Players. *J. Sport Rehabil.* **2014**, *23*, 88–94. [CrossRef]
20. Garrison, M.; Westrick, R.; Johnson, M.R.; Benenson, J. Association between the functional movement screen and injury development in college athletes. *Int. J. Sports Phys. Ther.* **2015**, *10*, 21–28.
21. Letafatkar, A.; Hadadnezhad, M.; Shojaedin, S.; Mohamadi, E. Relationship between functional movement screening score and history of injury. *Int. J. Sports Phys. Ther.* **2014**, *9*, 21–27. [PubMed]
22. Dossa, K.; Cashman, G.; Howitt, S.; West, B.; Murray, N. Can injury in major junior hockey players be predicted by a pre-season functional movement screen—A prospective cohort study. *J. Can. Chiropr. Assoc.* **2014**, *58*, 421–427. [PubMed]
23. Bardenett, S.M.; Micca, J.J.; De Noyelles, J.T.; Miller, S.D.; Jenk, D.T.; Brooks, G.S. Functional Movement Screen Normative Values and Validity in High School Athletes: Can the Fms™ be Used as a Predictor of Injury? *Int. J. Sports Phys. Ther.* **2015**, *10*, 303–308. [PubMed]
24. Dorrel, B.S.; Long, T.; Shaffe, S.; Myer, G.D. Evaluation of the Functional Movement Screen as an Injury Prediction Tool among Active Adult Populations: A Systematic Review and Meta-analysis. *Sports Health* **2015**, *7*, 532–537. [CrossRef] [PubMed]
25. Quatman-Yates, C.C.; Quatman, C.E.; Meszaros, A.J.; Paterno, M.V.; Hewett, T.E. A systematic review of sensorimotor function during adolescence: A developmental stage of increased motor awkwardness? *Br. J. Sports Med.* **2012**, *46*, 649–655. [CrossRef] [PubMed]
26. Štefan, L.; Sorić, M.; Devrnja, A.; Podnar, H.; Mišigoj-Duraković, M. Is school type associated with objectively measured physical activity in 15-year-olds? *Int. J. Environ. Res. Public Health* **2017**, *14*, 1417. [CrossRef] [PubMed]
27. Gulgin, H.; Hoogenboom, B. The Functional Movement screening (FMSTM): An Inter-rater Reliability Study between Raters of Varied Experience. *Int. J. Sports. Phys. Ther.* **2014**, *9*, 14–20.
28. Teyhen, D.S.; Shaffer, S.W.; Lorenson, C.L.; Halfpap, J.P.; Donofry, D.F.; Walker, M.J.; Dugan, J.L.; Childs, J.D. The Functional Movement Screen: A Reliability Study. *J. Orthop. Sports Phys. Ther.* **2012**, *42*, 530–540. [CrossRef]

29. Sterling, M.; Jull, G.; Wright, A. The effect of musculoskeletal pain on motor activity and control. *J. Pain* **2001**, *2*, 135–145. [CrossRef]
30. Bernard, J.; Bard, R.; Pujol, À.; Combey, A.; Boussard, D.; Begué, C.; Salghetti, A. Muscle assessment in healthy teenagers, Comparison with teenagers with low back pain. *Ann. Readapt. Med. Phys.* **2008**, *51*, 263–283. [CrossRef]
31. Jansson, A.; Saartok, T.; Werner, S.; Renstrom, P. General joint laxity in 1845 Swedish school children of different ages: Age and gender-specific distributions. *Acta Paediatr.* **2004**, *93*, 1202–1206. [CrossRef] [PubMed]
32. Gómez-Campos, R.; Andruske, C.L.; Arruda, M.; Sulla-Torres, J.; Pacheco-Carrillo, J.; Urra-Albornoz, C.; Cossio-bolaños, M. Normative data for handgrip strength in children and adolescents in the Maule Region, Chile: Evaluation based on chronological and biological age. *PLoS ONE* **2018**, *13*, e0201033. [CrossRef] [PubMed]
33. Shultz, S.J.; Nguyen, A.D.; Schmitz, R.J. Differences in Lower Extremity Anatomical and Postural Characteristics in Males and Females between Maturation Groups. *J. Orthop. Sports Phys. Ther.* **2008**, *38*, 137–149. [CrossRef] [PubMed]
34. Huseynov, A.; Zollikofer, C.P.; Coudyzer, W.; Gascho, D.; Kellenberger, C.; Hinzpeter, R.; De León, M.S.P. Developmental evidence for obstetric adaptation of the human female pelvis. *Proc. Natl. Acad. Sci. USA* **2016**, *113*, 5227–5232. [CrossRef] [PubMed]
35. Peterson, J.B.; Doan, J.; Bomar, J.D.; Wenger, D.R.; Pennock, A.T.; Upasani, V.V. Sex Differences in Cartilage Topography and Orientation of the Developing Acetabulum: Implications for Hip Preservation Surgery. *Clin. Orthop. Relat. Res.* **2015**, *473*, 2489–2494. [CrossRef] [PubMed]
36. Hooper, P.; Oak, S.R.; Lynch, T.S.; Ibrahim, G.; Goodwin, R.; Rosneck, J. Adolescent Femoroacetabular Impingement: Gender Differences in Hip Morphology. *Arthrosc. J. Arthrosc. Relat. Surg.* **2016**, *32*, 2495–2502. [CrossRef] [PubMed]
37. Slater, A.; Tiggemann, M. Gender differences in adolescent sport participation, teasing, self-objectification and body image concerns. *J. Adolesc.* **2011**, *34*, 455–463. [CrossRef]

Publisher's Note: MDPI stays neutral with regard to jurisdictional claims in published maps and institutional affiliations.

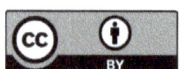

© 2020 by the authors. Licensee MDPI, Basel, Switzerland. This article is an open access article distributed under the terms and conditions of the Creative Commons Attribution (CC BY) license (http://creativecommons.org/licenses/by/4.0/).

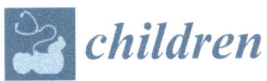

Article

Predicting Injury Status in Adolescent Dancers Involved in Different Dance Styles: A Prospective Study

Damir Sekulic [1,*], Dasa Prus [2], Ante Zevrnja [3], Mia Peric [1] and Petra Zaletel [2]

1. Faculty of Kinesiology, University of Split, 21000 Split, Croatia; mia.peric@kifst.hr
2. Faculty of Sport, University of Ljubljana, 1000 Ljubljana, Slovenia; dasa.prus@fsp.uni-lj.si (D.P.); petra.zaletel@fsp.uni-lj.si (P.Z.)
3. Clinical Hospital Split, 21000 Split, Croatia; antezevrnja17@gmail.com
* Correspondence: dado@kifst.hr

Received: 30 November 2020; Accepted: 15 December 2020; Published: 16 December 2020

Abstract: The positive effects of dance on health indices in youth are widely recognized, but participation in dance is accompanied with a certain risk of injury. This prospective study aimed to investigate injury occurrence and to evaluate the possible influences of specific predictors on the occurrence of musculoskeletal problems and injuries in adolescent dancers. Participants were 126 dancers (21 males; 11–18 years), who were competitors in the urban dance, rock and roll, and standard/Latin dance genres. Predictors included sociodemographic factors, anthropometric/body build indices, sport (dance) factors, and dynamic balance. The outcome variable was injury status, and this was evaluated by the Oslo Sports Trauma Research Centre Overuse Injury Questionnaire (OSTRC). Predictors were evaluated at baseline, and outcomes were continuously monitored during the study period of 3 months. During the study course, 53% of dancers reported the occurrence of a musculoskeletal problem/injury, and dancers suffered from an average of 0.72 injuries over the study period (95% CI: 0.28–1.41), giving a yearly injury rate of 280%. Gender and dance styles were not significantly related to the occurrence of injury. Higher risk for injury was evidenced in older and more experienced dancers. Dynamic balance, as measured by the Star Excursion Balance Test (SEBT), was a significant protective factor of injury occurrence, irrespective of age/experience in dance. Knowing the simplicity and applicability of the SEBT, continuous monitoring of dynamic balance in adolescent dancers is encouraged. In order to prevent the occurrence of musculoskeletal problems/injuries in youth dancers, we suggest the incorporation of specific interventions aimed at improving dynamic balance.

Keywords: musculoskeletal injury; sports; exercise; risk factors; protective factors

1. Introduction

The importance of participating in sufficient physical activity (PA) in childhood and adolescence and the benefits of PA on physical health, mental health, academic performance, and social well-being have been well proven [1–5]. However, the decrease in participation in PA in adolescence is recognized as a global problem, which is additionally important since a decrease in PA may extend into adult life [6–8]. Despite the fact that Slovenian children and adolescents are among the most physically active in the world, their levels of PA have decreased in recent years, and this problem is especially exacerbated during adolescence [9].

To prevent a decrease in PA, various interventional programs have been constructed to encourage children and adolescents to be more physically active [10,11]. Since such programs should be motivational and attractive, dance is a perfect tool, as it fulfils not only PA requirements but also enables the development of social skills and expressiveness in youth [12–14]. As some individuals begin to dance very early in their childhood, dance is a particularly suitable form of PA that can be continuously applied whether in a professional or recreational context, throughout a participant's lifetime [15–17].

However, as with any other PA, dance participation is accompanied by a certain risk of injury, even in youth [17–19]. Studies have reported that 20–84% of dancers have suffered from a musculoskeletal (MS) injury at least once in their career, and an even higher percentage (95%) have suffered from MS pain [18,20,21]. MS injuries vary by dance style, and by far the most common dancers to experience MS injuries are ballet dancers, followed by urban dancers (i.e., breakdance, hip-hop, locking, popping, house) and modern dancers [16,22,23].

Collectively, studies have confirmed higher injury rates in older dancers and/or shown a correlation between a dancer's age and the occurrence of injury [24]. Further, due to characteristics of the dance activity and specifics of artistic expression, anthropometric/body build indices are known to be associated with injury risk, with a higher risk of injury in dancers with longer body segments and more body fat [25]. Studies have also confirmed that a there is a higher risk for injury occurrence in female dancers than in their male peers, which is connected to the most commonly injured body location in dancers (the knee), whereby the larger Q-angle in females potentially translates into greater forces of the quadriceps being applied to the patella and encourages mal-tracking [26,27]. Finally, a recent study provided evidence of a possible influence of dynamic balance as a protective factor against injury occurrence in dance, which was explained by the connection between dynamic balance and a dancer's ability to sustain equilibrium by keeping their body over its base of support [17,28].

Irrespective of the well proven benefits of dance and the risks of participation in dance, only a few studies have exclusively examined youth dancers with regard to injury prevalence and factors of influence. In brief, US authors examined adolescent dancers (avg. age 15.3 y) at a liberal arts high school dance program over a one-year period (school year). Dancers self-reported 112 injuries (avg. 2.8 of self-reported injuries per dancer), and older age turned out to be the prevalent risk factor associated with self-reported injuries [24]. In a study of injury patterns in young, non-professional dancers, advanced age and increased exposure to dance (i.e., age) were also proven to be correlated with an increased prevalence of injury in girls (age 8–16 y) [29]. Meanwhile, there is an evident lack of studies that have prospectively examined factors associated with injury occurrence in youth dancers involved in different dance styles.

Therefore, the aim of this study was to prospectively analyze the injury occurrence in adolescent dancers involved in different dance styles (urban dance, standard/Latin dance, rock and roll) and to evaluate the possible factors influencing the occurrence of MS problems and injuries. Specifically, based on results of previous studies on different dance styles, we were particularly interested in anthropometric/body build indices, sociodemographic and dance factors, and dynamic balance as factors of possible influence on injury status in adolescent dancers. We hypothesized that the studied factors significantly influence the injury status of adolescent dancers.

2. Materials and Methods

2.1. Participants and Design

A total of 126 young dancers (21 males) involved in urban dance (breakdance, hip-hop, locking, popping, house; $n = 99$), rock and roll ($n = 14$), and standard and Latin-American dance ($n = 13$) all aged 11–18 years (mean age 15.66 ± 1.57) from Slovenia participated in the present study. Participants were selected on the basis of their status in dance sport, and all participants should be regular competitors at national and international levels under the auspices of the Slovenian Dance Association (SDA) and the International Dance Organization at the study baseline. The participants had an average of 7.8 ± 2.78 years of dance experience and trained for 7.09 ± 4.56 h per week at their respective dance schools. Based on (i) a previously evidenced injury occurrence of 10% [17], (ii) a population sample of 621 registered adolescent dancers in Slovenia for the studied year, (iii) margin of error of 0.05, and (iv) confidence level of 0.95, the required sample size for this investigation was calculated to be 114 participants (calculated by Statistica, Tibco Software Inc., Palo Alto, CA, USA)

In 2018, when the study was done, there were 23 dance teams/schools with registered adolescent dancers in Slovenia. All schools were invited to participate in the study by the SDA, and dancers were informed about the study's aims, protocol, potential benefits, and risks. The participants were asked to provide consent from their parents, and participation was voluntary and anonymous. Dancers were qualified for inclusion if they were (i) minors (18 years or younger at the end of the study—see later for design), (ii) officially registered as a competition participant in the International Dance Organization, and (iii) participating in at least two dance trainings per week. Exclusion criteria included age of 18+ at the end of the study, non-regular participation in dance training (less than two dance trainings per week as defined by main coach), and injury/sickness during the baseline testing (see later for details on testing). Participants willing to be enrolled in the study were invited to screening at the Institute of Sport (University of Ljubljana, Faculty of Sport, Ljubljana, Slovenia). Involvement in the research was voluntary, and participants' personal data were protected with an identification code, known only to the main/head researcher. The study protocol was approved by the Ethics Committee of the University of Ljubljana, Faculty of Sport, Ljubljana, Slovenia (Ref. number: 1175/2017). This prospective study included testing, which was done at baseline and during a follow-up period. Baseline testing of predictors (see later for details) was done in December 2018–January 2019, and follow-up testing was performed continuously over a period of 3 months after baseline and included an analysis of outcome.

2.2. Variables

Predictors included sociodemographic characteristics, anthropometric indices, dance factors, and dynamic balance (predictors). The outcome variable in this study was injury status.

2.2.1. Sociodemographic and Dance Factors

Sociodemographic variables included age and gender. For the dance factors, dancers were asked about their (i) dance style (urban, standard/Latin (S/L), or rock and roll (RNR)), (ii) experience in dance (in years), (iii) age when they started to practice (later transformed into years of experience in dance), (iv) number of weekly training sessions, and (v) hours of weekly training.

2.2.2. Anthropometric and Body-Built Indices

Anthropometrics included (i) body height (in 0.5 cm) and (ii) body mass (in 0.1 kg), both measured with standardized techniques and calibrated equipment and (iii) calculated body mass index (BMI; in kg/m^2) and body composition indices (body fat percentage (BF%), and lean body mass (kg). Body composition was measured by bioelectrical impedance analysis with the InBody 720 Tetrapolar 8-Point Tactile Electrode System (Biospace Co. Ltd., Seoul, Korea) [30,31].

2.2.3. Dynamic Balance

The Star Excursion Balance Test (SEBT), a functional screening tool, was used to measure balance performance in dancers. The test was designed to assess dynamic lower extremity balance, monitor rehabilitation progress, screen for deficits in dynamic postural control due to MS injuries, and identify athletes at high risk for lower limb injuries [32]. Performance of the test requires good balance, flexibility, strength, and coordination of the lower extremities. Although some authors have reported contradictory results regarding the accuracy of the SEBT test and its modifications as a predictor of an athlete's risk of injury, the majority of recent studies have confirmed SEBT as one of the most prominent non-equipment screening tools to measure dynamic balance of the lower extremities [33]. SEBT has previously been shown to be a reliable measure and has been validated for use as a dynamic test for predicting the risk of lower limb injury [33]. Furthermore, the results of a recent systematic review showed that the SEBT has great inter- and intra-rater reliability [34]. The SEBT consists of eight-line grids, extending from the center point, with 45 degree angles between them. Every direction poses different demands and combinations regarding each motor ability in the frontal, sagittal, and transverse planes. Grids were taped on the floor with adhesive tape marked with centimeters. Individual verbal instructions and a demonstration were given to each participant by the same examiner, who then supervised the proper execution of the test. The participants took a unilateral position, with the stance foot in the center of the grid. Dancers had to reach down all of the marked lines as far as possible, using the non-stance leg, and then return with their reach leg back to the center of the grid, while maintaining a unilateral position. Dancers kept their hands flexed at the iliac crest throughout the test protocol. A result was not considered if (i) the dancer was not able to maintain the single-leg stance, (ii) the dancer changed the position of the foot during the trial (lifted their heel or toes off the floor, rotated the foot), (iii) the dancer's weight was transferred onto the reaching foot, (iv) the dancer's hands did not remain on their hips, or (v) the dancer was not able to firmly maintain the start and return position. The reaching distances were measured to centimeter accuracy and normalized to the % leg length of the participants. The variables observed in this investigation included the normalized SEBT performance when participants were standing on their right leg (R1–R8) and left leg (L1–L8). All dancers were evaluated by same examiner in the same facility (Faculty of Sport, Ljubljana, Slovenia). Measurement of the SEBT is presented in Figure 1.

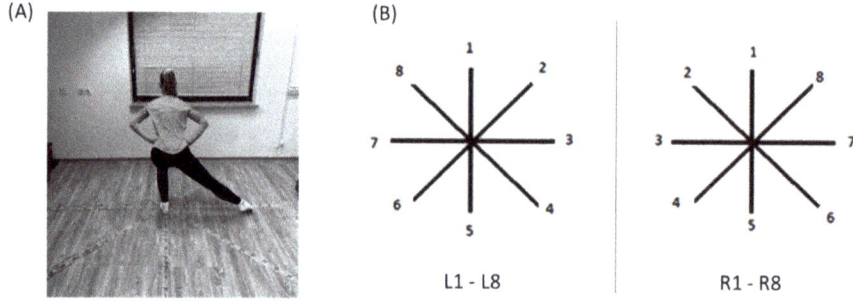

Figure 1. Execution of the Star Excursion Balance Test (**A**), and scoring while standing on the left leg (L1–L8) and while standing on the right leg (R1–R8) (**B**).

2.2.4. Injury Status

Injuries were recorded using the Oslo Sports Trauma Research Center Overuse Injury Questionnaire (OSTRC) [35]. Dancers responded to the OSTRC at baseline and prospectively once per week over the course of the study. At baseline, participants were personally asked about injury occurrence in the 3 month period before the testing. A digital form of the questionnaire was sent to participants by e-mail once a week. Additional individual reminders were sent to participants who did not provide any data for the preceding week. The outcome of this study was the incidence of MS problems and injuries that occurred during the study course in four body regions: ankle, knee, back, and shoulder. Each answer in the OSTRC corresponds to a score. For each question (body location), a score between 0 and 25 is given, and a theoretical score (sum) ranging from 0 to 100 is calculated for four body regions. Reported scores of >39 were classified as the occurrence of MS injury (MSI; for the purpose of multinomial regression, they were later numerically scored as "2"). The presence of a MS problem (MSP) was considered if the participant scored anything higher than the lowest grade on each question (scored as "1" in regression calculation). Finally, if the participant reported a score of "zero" for all questions, the absence of any problem/injury was recorded (scored as "0" later in the regression calculation).

2.3. Data Analysis

In the first phase of statistical analysis, all variables were checked for the normality of distribution by the Kolmogorov–Smirnov test. Descriptive statistics calculated for variables found to be normally distributed included the means and standard deviations; otherwise, frequencies (F) and percentages (%) are reported. Injury rates are reported as the total number of injuries per studied period and the number of injuries relative to hours of exposure (dance hours; with 95% CI for Poisson rates). For these data, and irrespective of the OSTRC specific graduation, in the following text, all scores higher than minimum (zero) are collectively considered as an "injury", if not specified otherwise.

The differences in studied categorical variables were evaluated by the chi-square test. The analysis of variance (ANOVA) was calculated in order to identify differences between/among groups, for parametric/normally distributed variables, with additional calculation of the Welch's p due to unequal sample size of groups when comparison among dance styles was done.

The associations between studied predictors and outcomes (MS problem/injury) were evaluated by a univariate multinomial regression calculation using multinomial criteria based on the categorized OSTRC scale (0 = absence of MS problem/injury, 1 = MS problem, 2 = MS injury), with the absence of a problem/injury being the referent value in the multinomial regression calculation. Authors were of the opinion that usage of the multinomial regression will allow clear identification of the factors associated with MS problem and MS injury, especially knowing the differences in subjective perception of pain as an indicator of MS problem/injury. The odds ratio (OR) with the corresponding 95% confidence interval (95% CI) was reported. Multinomial regression calculations included nonadjusted regression correlations and correlations adjusted for gender, age, and dance style (Model 1). Statistica ver. 13.5 (Tibco Inc., Palo Alto, CA, USA) was used for all analyses, and a significance level of $p < 0.05$ was applied.

3. Results

During the study period (November/December 2018–March/April 2019), 59 dancers (47%) reported no MS injury/problem, 43% (54 dancers) reported an MS problem, and 10% (13 dancers) reported an MS injury (Figure 2). When compared across dance styles, no significant differences were obtained (Chi square = 1.51, $p = 0.84$). Altogether, 67 dancers (53%) reported at least one injury/problem, a prevalence of 39%. Multiple injuries/problems were reported by 10% of dancers. Over approximately 7050 h of dance and 91 injuries/problems occurred in total (95% CI: 73–111).

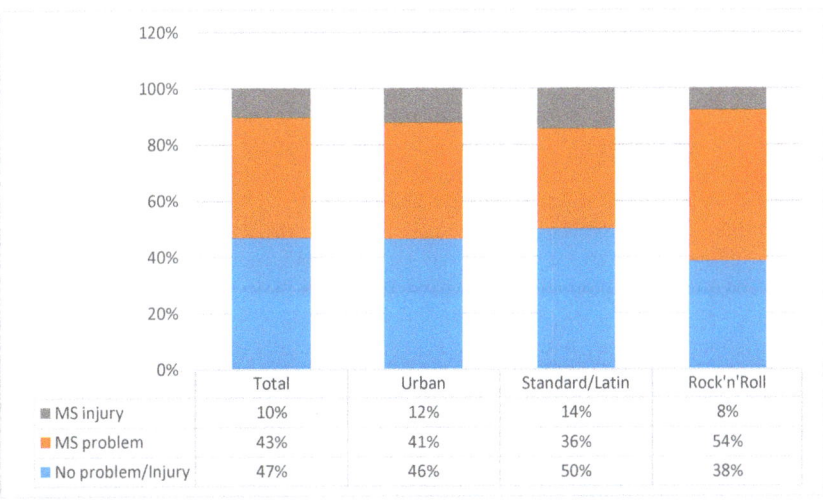

Figure 2. Prevalence of the musculoskeletal (MS) problems and injures in adolescent dancers.

The lowest prevalence of injury occurred in females involved in S/L, with 71% of dancers experiencing no problem/injury over the study course. On the other hand, males involved in urban dances experienced highest rates of injury (18%) with additional 45% who experienced some kind of MS problem over the course of the study. The most evident difference between males and females was evidenced for standard/Latin dances, where males reported more MS problems/injury than females (71% females and 29% males reported no MS problem/injury) (Figure 3).

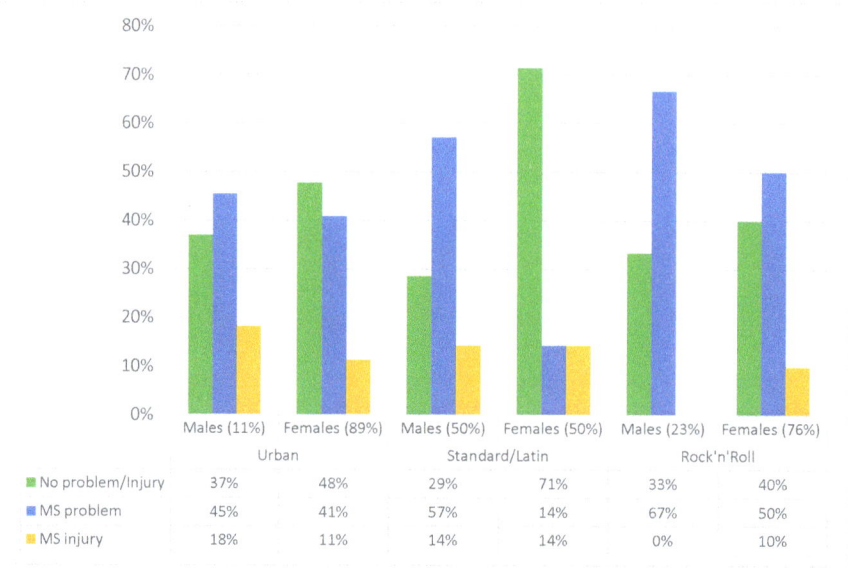

Figure 3. Prevalence of the musculoskeletal (MS) problems and injuries in adolescent dancers according to gender for studied dance styles.

On average, each dancer suffered from 0.72 injuries over the study period (95% CI: 0.28–1.41) with similar rates of occurrence for both genders (0.67 (95% CI: 0.51–0.85) and 0.78 (95% CI: 0.61–0.97) in females and males, respectively), with no significant difference between genders (MW = 1.22, p = 0.21), a rate of 2.88 injuries per dancer per year.

Differences in the studied predictors among dance styles are shown in Table 1. The S/L dancers had been involved in dance for the shortest amount of time, but they participated in more training hours than the RNR and urban dancers did. A significant difference in BF% between individuals involved in different dance styles was shown, with SL dancers being the leanest. Differences in SBT were shown for 10 of 16 variables, and in all cases urban dancers had the lowest performance, with no significant differences between RNR and S/L dancers.

For non-adjusted regression, the higher odds for the occurrence of MS injury were shown for older dancers (OR = 1.51, 95% CI: 1.11–2.04) and for those who had had a longer career in dance (OR = 1.31, 95% CI: 1.04–1.67). Dancers with more experience in dance were at a greater risk for reporting an MS problem (OR = 1.17, 95% CI 1.04–1.32) or MS injury (OR = 1.17, 95% CI: 1.01–1.38). Gender, dance style, and anthropometric/body build indices did not significantly influence the occurrence of MS problem/injury. Several SEBT variables were correlated with MS injury/problem, with lower odds for MS injury/problem occurring in dancers who achieved better SEBT normalized scores. Namely, significant influences of dynamic balance on the occurrence of an MS problem/injury were recorded for R3 (OR (95% CI); MS injury: OR = 0.95 (0.91–0.99)), R4 (MS problem: 0.98 (0.96–0.99); MS injury: 0.97 (0.95–0.99)), R5 (MS problem: 0.98 (0.96–0.99); MS injury: 0.97 (0.95–0.99)), R6 (MS problem: 0.98 (0.96–0.99)), R7 (MS problem: 0.98 (0.96–0.99)), L3 (MS problem: 0.98 (0.95–0.99)), L5 (MS problem: 0.98

(0.97–0.99); MS injury: 0.98 (0.95–0.99)), L6 (MS problem: 0.98 (0.96–0.99); MS injury: 0.97 (0.95–0.99)), L7 (MS problem: 0.97 (0.95–0.99)), and L8 (MS problem: 0.96 (0.92–0.99)) (Table 2).

Table 1. Descriptive statistics (presented as means ± standard deviations) and differences between dance styles in studied variables (ANOVA with additional Welch's p calculation).

	Urban Dances	Standard/Latin Dances	Rock and Roll	ANOVA		Welch's p
	(n = 99)	(n = 14)	(n = 13)	F Test	p	
Age (years)	15.8 ± 1.4	15.25 ± 1.96	15.57 ± 1.66	1.42	0.241	0.031
Started with dance (years)	7.77 ± 2.8	9.3 ± 2.7	7.52 ± 3.25	3.08	0.052	0.294
Involvement in dance (years)	8.11 ± 2.65	6 ± 2.65	8.29 ± 2.72	6.47	0.001	0.001
Trainings per week (f)	3.42 ± 0.87	5.57 ± 1.53	5.1 ± 0.89	63.09	0.001	0.001
Hours of training per week (h)	5.41 ± 1.77	17.91 ± 6.13	11.14 ± 2.39	205.47	0.001	0.001
Body height (cm)	165.85 ± 6.33	167.23 ± 9.97	166.91 ± 10.93	0.44	0.651	0.832
Body mass (kg)	58.92 ± 7.01	55 ± 11.38	58.68 ± 13.33	2.01	0.143	0.082
Body fat (%)	21.89 ± 6.51	12.09 ± 5.26	15.51 ± 5.63	29.52	0.001	0.001
Lean body mass (%)	25.34 ± 3.39	26.91 ± 6.65	27.54 ± 6.95	2.97	0.052	0.567
Body mass index (kg/m^2)	21.43 ± 2.44	19.45 ± 2.1	20.83 ± 2.58	6.71	0.001	0.001
R1 (SEBT result/leg length)	83.86 ± 9.61	85.35 ± 5.88	83.29 ± 6.6	0.32	0.721	0.022
R2 (SEBT result/leg length)	89.25 ± 12.36	95.8 ± 12.79	92.21 ± 6.38	3.00	0.052	0.031
R3 (SEBT result/leg length)	100.23 ± 14.08	124.77 ± 23.14	111.32 ± 12.83	24.83	0.001	0.001
R4 (SEBT result/leg length)	105.72 ± 16.31	128.73 ± 20.3	130.17 ± 14.08	31.70	0.001	0.001
R5 (SEBT result/leg length)	106.1 ± 16.82	132.11 ± 19.63	134.72 ± 20.57	37.03	0.001	0.001
R6 (SEBT result/leg length)	100.07 ± 16.68	125.27 ± 22.6	127.35 ± 23.22	31.42	0.001	0.001
R7 (SEBT result/leg length)	89.04 ± 15.75	114.04 ± 22.76	106.71 ± 16.45	25.78	0.001	0.001
R8 (SEBT result/leg length)	74.84 ± 10.02	75.6 ± 11.36	75.23 ± 5.37	0.06	0.94	0.323
L1 (SEBT result/leg length)	83.52 ± 9.96	81.72 ± 5.42	81.25 ± 7.67	0.75	0.471	0.541
L2 (SEBT result/leg length)	89.82 ± 10.04	90.99 ± 8.3	90.85 ± 7.55	0.20	0.823	0.289
L3 (SEBT result/leg length)	99.2 ± 14.65	116.9 ± 20.78	116.79 ± 13.3	19.97	0.001	0.001
L4 (SEBT result/leg length)	107.38 ± 16.26	129.77 ± 20.22	130.52 ± 14.23	28.69	0.001	0.001
L5 (SEBT result/leg length)	106.71 ± 17.92	132.19 ± 21.65	135.68 ± 17.47	33.52	0.001	0.001
L6 (SEBT result/leg length)	100.57 ± 17.57	127.77 ± 23.2	125.65 ± 19.59	30.13	0.001	0.001
L7 (SEBT result/leg length)	90.12 ± 14.92	110.84 ± 23.65	107.39 ± 17.89	20.16	0.001	0.001
L8 (SEBT result/leg length)	74.48 ± 11.99	77.95 ± 10.23	77.13 ± 13.53	1.02	0.364	0.046

R1–R8—normalized result on Star Excursion Balance Test (SEBT) while standing on the right leg in eight directions; L1–L8—normalized result on Star Excursion Balance Test (SEBT) while standing on the left leg.

Table 2. Correlates of musculoskeletal problems and injury in adolescent dancers; results are given as OR (95% CI).

	Model 0 (Nonadjusted)		Model 1 (Adjusted for Dance Style, Age, and Gender)	
	MS Problem	MS Injury	MS Problem	MS Injury
Male gender	1.57 (0.58–4.21)	1.05 (0.39–2.76)		
Age (years)	1.09 (0.89–1.33)	1.51 (1.11–2.04)		
Involvement in dance (years)	1.05 (0.91–1.20)	1.31 (1.04–1.66)	1.01 (0.88–1.23)	1.11 (0.91–1.51)
Training per week (hours)	1.05 (0.93–1.25)	1.00 (0.87–1.17)	1.03 (0.91–1.27)	1.01 (0.85–1.20)
Body height (cm)	1.00 (0.97–1.05)	0.99 (0.94–1.05)	1.00 (0.96–1.07)	1.00 (0.93–1.06)
Body mass (kg)	1.02 (0.98–1.06)	1.02 (0.97–1.07)	1.01 (0.96–1.08)	1.01 (0.96–1.08)
Body fat (%)	1.00 (0.97–1.05)	1.05 (0.97–1.15)	1.01 (0.98–1.08)	1.06 (0.98–1.17)
Lean body mass (kg)	1.01 (0.95–1.08)	0.99 (0.92–1.08)	1.02 (0.94–1.09)	0.99 (0.91–1.10)
Body mass index (kg/m^2)	0.97 (0.83–1.14)	0.98 (0.81–1.21)	0.95 (0.81–1.15)	0.95 (0.80–1.23)
R1 (SEBT result/leg length)	0.97 (0.92–1.03)	0.93 (0.86–1.00)	0.98 (0.90–1.05)	0.93 (0.86–1.00)
R2 (SEBT result/leg length)	0.99 (0.95–1.03)	0.94 (0.89–1.01)	1.00 (0.92–1.05)	0.96 (0.87–1.04)
R3 (SEBT result/leg length)	0.99 (0.97–1.01)	0.95 (0.91–0.99)	0.98 (0.94–1.01)	0.96 (0.92–0.99)
R4 (SEBT result/leg length)	0.98 (0.96–0.99)	0.97 (0.95–0.99)	0.99 (0.94–1.03)	0.98 (0.92 1.03)
R5 (SEBT result/leg length)	0.98 (0.96–0.99)	0.97 (0.95–0.99)	0.99 (0.94–1.02)	0.98 (0.93–1.03)
R6 (SEBT result/leg length)	0.98 (0.97–0.99)	0.98 (0.96–1.01)	0.99 (0.95–1.04)	0.98 (0.94–1.02)
R7 (SEBT result/leg length)	0.98 (0.96–0.99)	0.99 (0.96–1.01)	0.97 (0.94–1.01)	0.98 (0.95–1.02)
R8 (SEBT result/leg length)	0.96 (0.93–1.01)	1.01 (0.96–1.06)	0.98 (0.92–1.04)	1.00 (0.95–1.06)

Table 2. *Cont.*

	Model 0 (Nonadjusted)		Model 1 (Adjusted for Dance Style, Age, and Gender)	
	MS Problem	MS Injury	MS Problem	MS Injury
L1 (SEBT result/leg length)	0.98 (0.93–1.02)	0.98 (0.93–1.03)	0.99 (0.94–1.05)	1.00 (0.94–1.04)
L2 (SEBT result/leg length)	0.99 (0.95–1.03)	0.99 (0.94–1.04)	0.99 (0.95–1.04)	0.99 (0.94–1.05)
L3 (SEBT result/leg length)	0.98 (0.96–0.99)	0.98 (0.96–1.01)	0.98 (0.95–0.99)	0.98 (0.95–1.02)
L4 (SEBT result/leg length)	0.98 (0.97–1.01)	0.98 (0.96–1.01)	0.99 (0.97–1.02)	1.00 (0.97–1.03)
L5 (SEBT result/leg length)	0.98 (0.97–0.99)	0.98 (0.95–0.99)	0.99 (0.97–1.02)	1.00 (0.95–1.05)
L6 (SEBT result/leg length)	0.98 (0.96–0.99)	0.97 (0.95–0.99)	0.98 (0.96–0.99)	0.97 (0.95–0.99)
L7 (SEBT result/leg length)	0.97 (0.95–0.99)	0.98 (0.95–1.01)	0.98 (0.95–1.01)	0.99 (0.95–1.03)
L8 (SEBT result/leg length)	0.96 (0.92–0.99)	0.97 (0.93–1.01)	0.97 (0.93–0.99)	0.98 (0.92–1.03)

R1–R8—normalized result on Star Excursion Balance Test (SEBT) while standing on the right leg in eight directions; L1–L8—normalized result on Star Excursion Balance Test (SEBT) while standing on the left leg.

In order to statistically control the possible influences of age, gender, and dancing experience, multinomial regressions were calculated between SEBT measures, including age, gender, and dance style as confounding factors (i.e., age was a stronger predictor of an MS problem/injury than experience in dance (please see previous results), while age and dance experience were shown to be naturally correlated). Generally, even for these calculations, a similar protective influence of dynamic balance on MS problem/injury occurrence was shown, although not all variables found to be significantly correlated with the occurrence of an MS problem/injury in the "crude" model were significantly associated with the outcome in the regression model, which controlled for confounding factors (Model 1). Specifically, Model 1 showed that there was a lower likelihood of an MS problem/injury occurring for dancers who achieved better scores for R3 (OR (95% CI); MS injury: 0.96 (0.92–0.99)), L3 (MS problem: 0.98 (0.95–0.99)), L6 (MS problem: 0.98 (0.96–0.99); MS injury: 0.97 (0.95–0.99)), and L8 (MS problem: 0.97 (0.93–0.99)) (Table 2).

4. Discussion

With regard to the study's aims, there are several important findings. First, the results provided no evidence of gender being a significant factor of influence on injury status. Next, a higher risk for MS injury/problem was found for older and more experienced adolescent dancers. Finally, dynamic balance was an important protective factor against MS problems/injury, irrespective of a participant's age. Thus, the results partially support our initial study hypothesis.

4.1. Gender and Injury Occurrence

The injury rate of 2.8 injuries per year per dancer (280%) is somewhat lower than that presented in a recent study on Slovenian dancers, where the authors reported an injury rate of 310% [17]. However, this is not surprising since we studied younger dancers, and the risk of injury increases with age and exposure to dance [22]. Actually, the association between age and injury occurrence was confirmed in our study and will be discussed later.

We found no significant influence of gender on injury risk. This is in certain disagreement with previous reports that mostly identified a higher risk for injury among female dancers. For example, an international study revealed that females had a significantly higher median injury incidence than males and confirmed that there were gender differences regarding reported traumatic injuries, with a higher incidence of traumatic injuries occurring in females (74.6%) than males (46.7%) [27]. Supportively, another study showed that female dancers have a higher injury risk than their male counterparts [26]. Collectively, this was explained as being due to (i) the knee being the most commonly injured location, and (ii) the larger Q-angle in females that potentially translates into a greater force of the quadriceps being applied to the patella, as well as a greater likelihood for mal-tracking [26]

However, to the best of our knowledge, this is one of the first studies which examined gender as a possible factor of injury exclusively in adolescent dancers. This probably explains the discrepancy between our findings and those of previous studies where female dancers were reported to have a greater injury risk than their male peers [26,27]. We must highlight the fact that those studies involved older adolescents and adult dancers. More comparable to our study and therefore our findings is a Brazilian study of pre-professional male and female dancers (17 ± 4.44 years of age), where the authors noted no significant effect of gender on injury incidence [36]. Collectively, it seems that gender differences in injury prevalence (e.g., higher injury rate in females) are more apparent in adult than in youth dancers. However, we must note that our analysis was performed on the sample as a whole (i.e., regardless of dance style); therefore, dance-style-specific analyses are necessary. This is particularly evident if we take a closer look on gender differences in some dance styles. Specifically, in our study males involved in standard/Latin dances were more injured than their female partners. It almost certainly points to specific mechanisms of MS problem/injury for those athletes, and it deserves more attention in future investigations.

4.2. Age and Dance Factors as Predictors of Injury

It has already been reported that the age of a dancer can correlate with injury occurrence and risk of injury [19]. However, previous studies where injury risk was shown to increase with age regularly observed dancers with a greater age span and/or included adult dancers [37]. Meanwhile, the results of our study identified age as an important risk factor for injury occurrence, even among adolescent dancers. Our results also clearly point that an association between age and injury risk should actually be contextualized through the positive association of experience in dance (exposure to dance) and injury risk (e.g., higher injury risk occurs in dancers who have been exposed to dance for a longer period of time). Due to differences in the characteristics of samples (i.e., adolescent dancers in our study and adult dancers in previous studies), a comparison is not straightforward. Still, we can make some assumptions based on previous research findings.

Mechanical overload and excessive use, which increase with age and career length, are the most commonly reported mechanisms of injury [38]. Consequently, it is logical that more mature and experienced dancers have had greater exposure to repetitive movement patterns and are therefore at a higher risk of overload and consequent injury. In addition, greater involvement in (any) sport implies (i) a greater intensity of training and (ii) increased weekly training exposure [24,37,39]. Since injury occurs when the forces are applied to body tissues (i.e., bones, muscles) exceed the capacity of the tissue to tolerate the applied forces, increased intensity and volume of training are natural risk factors for injury occurrence [28].

Furthermore, authors investigating the prevalence and risk of MS injuries among professional dancers pointed out that with greater exposure to repetitive movement structures, functional anomalies begin to appear in dancers, leading to the adaptation of dance technique, resulting in worsened force transmission and the occurrence of microtrauma [40]. In support of this, the number of injuries per dancer is higher in professional dancers than in recreational dancers, indicating that greater dance exposure and higher technical demands correspond to an increase in risk for injury occurrence [41,42]. Currently, we are not able to identify which of the discussed factors related to age and experience in dance influence injury occurrence to the greatest extent, but some explanations are offered in the subsequent text, where we discuss the influence of balance capacity on injury occurrence.

In this study we observed different dance styles, and analyses indicated no significant influence of dance style on injury occurrence. This study is one of the first ones where injury occurrence was compared across different dance disciplines; therefore, we are not able to compare our results with those previously reported. However, from the authors' perspective, it is possible that injury occurrence does not vary across dance styles. On the other hand, it is almost certain that dancers involved in different dance styles suffer from different types of injury and/or injured different body locations [16,21,43], which should be explored more in detail in the future.

4.3. Balance and Injury Occurrence

Balance is considered to be an important contributing factor to injury occurrence in sport, although not all studies have confirmed the predictive value of balance capacity on injury occurrence in athletes [28,33,44,45]. For example, balance status, as measured by the Y-balance test (a simplified version of the Star Excursion test considered in this study), was found to be predictive of injury occurrence in high school basketball players [46]. Performance in the Y-balance test was also shown to be a risk factor for injury occurrence in division I athletes [47]. Interestingly, although theoretically, balance may be associated with injury occurrence in dance, and studies have rarely examined this issue. Most probably, the issue of reliability of balance testing and the fact that balance testing is relatively time consuming (in comparison to other tests of conditioning capacities) have resulted in little empirical evidence about any association between balance and injury in dance.

To the best of our knowledge, only one very recent study has confirmed the importance of balance status in the prediction of injury occurrence in dance [17]. In brief, the study, which involved 129 competitive hip hop dancers (17.95 ± 4.15 years of age), examined predictors of injury, and a higher injury risk was shown among dancers who attained poorer scores on the explicit SEBT variables, irrespective of previous injury status. However, in the cited study, there was a certain possibility that the variation in participants' age may have influenced both balance and injury status. Therefore, our results where balance was found to be a significant predictor of injury occurrence in adolescent dancers are novel, to some extent.

Indeed, the correlation between balance and the occurrence of an MS problem/injury in adolescent dancers is one of the important findings in this study. In brief, dancers who were shown to have better dynamic balance on the SEBT test were less likely to experience a lower extremity injury. In presenting this mechanism for the balance–injury relationship, it is important to highlight that balance is actually the ability to achieve a state of equilibrium by maintaining the body's center of gravity over its base of support [28]. At the same time, injury results when the load applied to a structure (i.e., tissue) exceeds the capacity of the structure to sustain the load. Consequently, there are two mechanisms that can reduce the risk of injury: (i) increasing the ability of the structure to sustain the load (i.e., by strengthening the structure), and (ii) reducing the load applied to the structure [28]. Our results actually support the later mechanisms (i.e., a better balance capacity reduces the load applied to a dancer's body structures).

Superior balance indicates better joint stability and accentuates superior neuromuscular mechanisms responsible for the co-contraction of agonists and antagonists. It actually means that dancers with better balance are more capable of achieving equilibrium and maintaining their center of gravity over the base of support [28]. In most dance forms, the base of support is the dancer's foot, which naturally explains the here-established relationship between better balance and lower injury risk. However, it is crucial to note that the importance of balance in injury prevention seems to overcome even the previously discussed negative influence of age on injury risk in adolescent dancers. Specifically, the logistic regression analysis with balance and age as potential predictors only showed balance measured by the SEBT as a significant predictor of injury risk. Therefore, it appears that improvement in balance can decrease the risk of injury, even in those adolescent dancers whose careers last longer (i.e., older and/or more experienced dancers).

From our perspective, the explanation for our findings concerns the characteristics of dance training and competition. Namely, in all dance styles and forms, dance routines and choreography become more demanding (i.e., stressful) as the age/experience of a dancer increases [43]. The application of increased acute stress to the locomotor system (i.e., due to higher and more frequent jumps, repeated high-intensity efforts), together with more complex choreography increases the overall physiological demands of dancing, altogether resulting in a higher risk of injury occurrence. At the same time, having a superior balance capacity decreases the amount of stress applied to the body, irrespective of all specified risk factors, which occur as a result of higher dancing demands and, consequently, higher forces being applied to body structures (i.e., bones, muscles, tendons). Based on our results, the increased physiological demands of dance training and competition, known to be regular consequences of advanced dance experience, should be considered as factors with less influence on injury risk than inferior dynamic balance.

Additional (supplementary) balance training aimed at the prevention and rehabilitation of MS injuries, as well as improving sport performance, have become increasingly popular in sports [48,49]. Specific equipment has constantly been developed and is used in this type of training (i.e., balance balls, semicircular platforms, slack line, different types of balance platforms, rotator discs). Collectively, various exercise modalities are confirmed to be effective in improvement of dynamic balance in youth, even those involved in competitive sports [50,51]. Literature suggests that positive effects may be expected from relatively short training sessions (4–15 min of workout per session), performed twice per week, while largest effects may be expected after 12 weeks of training, resulting in 24–36 training sessions in total [51]. Therefore, selected balance exercises can be elegantly included as a part of warm-up session several times per week, assuring the low-cost, and effective stimuli are aimed at improving the dynamic balance, even in youth dancers.

4.4. Limitations and Strengths

There are several limitations of this study. First, we must highlight the unequal number of dancers participating in the different styles. Therefore, although the analyses performed did not indicate a significant influence of dance style on injury occurrence, it is still possible that the results are not equally generalizable to all studied dance styles. Second, there is a certain possibility that balance status was actually altered by some indices not examined in this study. Next, we certainly did not observe all factors potentially related to injury occurrence, such as biological age, motor competence, conditioning status, etc. Therefore, in future studies, special attention should be paid to other indices of a dancer's status and their influences on injury occurrence. In addition, the outcome was measured using the OSTRC, and this measurement tool examines injury occurrence at four body sites. On the other hand, it is possible that dancers suffered from specific injuries at other locations (i.e., wrist, neck).

To the best of our knowledge, this is one of the first studies to examine injury occurrence and factors associated with injury occurrence exclusively in adolescent dancers involved in the most popular dance styles. The study used a low-cost and applicable measurement tool for the evaluation of balance status. Since we found a significant influence of balance, as measured by the SEBT, our results are applicable for various circumstances. Next, all participants were measured in the same facility by experienced evaluators. Finally, the prospective nature of the study and the consequent lack of recall bias are important strengths of the investigation.

5. Conclusions

This study provides evidence of the negative influences of age and experience on injury occurrence among adolescent dancers. This is a logical consequence of greater sport demands (as a result of increased complexity in dancing routines and choreography) and a higher volume of training. Therefore, even in youth dancers, in order to prevent injury, special attention should be placed on more experienced dancers.

Higher risk for injury was found in dancers with lower results in the SEBT. While this testing protocol is simple, reliable, cheap, and applicable in different circumstances, we suggest that regular screening of dynamic balance in dancers should occur. This will allow the identification of dancers with a potential risk for injury occurrence.

Analyses performed in this investigation showed that dynamic balance is a more important predictor of injury occurrence than age (experience in dance). Therefore, it is expected that improvement in balance could diminish the risk of injury in dancers, irrespective of their age/experience. In order to achieve a stable position during choreographed movements, dancers must continually improve their balance and thus reduce their injury risk. Collectively, we suggest that specific interventions/training aimed at the improvement of dynamic balance are important components of injury prevention for adolescent dancers.

Author Contributions: Data curation, D.P. and P.Z.; Formal analysis, D.S.; Investigation, D.P., M.P. and P.Z.; Methodology, D.S., A.Z., M.P. and P.Z.; Writing-original draft, D.S., A.Z. and M.P.; Writing-review & editing, D.P. All authors have read and agreed to the published version of the manuscript.

Funding: This research received no external funding.

Acknowledgments: Authors are grateful to Slovenian Dance Federation. Special thanks goes to all dancers who voluntary participated in the research.

Conflicts of Interest: The authors declare no conflict of interest.

References

1. Xiang, M.; Gu, X.; Zhang, X.; Moss, S.; Huang, C.; Nelson, L.P.; Zhang, T. Psychosocial mechanism of adolescents' depression: A dose-response relation with physical activity. *Children* **2020**, *7*, 37. [CrossRef] [PubMed]
2. Goh, T.L.; Leong, C.H.; Brusseau, T.A.; Hannon, J. Children's physical activity levels following participation in a classroom-based physical activity curriculum. *Children* **2019**, *6*, 76. [CrossRef] [PubMed]
3. Granger, E.; Di Nardo, F.; Harrison, A.; Patterson, L.; Holmes, R.; Verma, A. A systematic review of the relationship of physical activity and health status in adolescents. *Eur. J. Public Health* **2017**, *27*, 100–106. [CrossRef] [PubMed]
4. Lee, J.; Zhang, T.; Chu, T.L.A.; Gu, X. Effects of a need-supportive motor skill intervention on children's motor skill competence and physical activity. *Children* **2020**, *7*, 21. [CrossRef] [PubMed]
5. Moral-Garcia, J.E.; Agraso-Lopez, A.D.; Ramos-Morcillo, A.J.; Jimenez, A.; Jimenez-Eguizabal, A. The influence of physical activity, diet, weight status and substance abuse on students' self-perceived health. *Int. J. Environ. Res. Public Health* **2020**, *17*, 1387. [CrossRef] [PubMed]
6. Guthold, R.; Stevens, G.A.; Riley, L.M.; Bull, F.C. Global trends in insufficient physical activity among adolescents: A pooled analysis of 298 population-based surveys with 1.6 million participants. *Lancet Child Adolesc. Health* **2020**, *4*, 23–35. [CrossRef]
7. Llewellyn, A.; Simmonds, M.; Owen, C.G.; Woolacott, N. Childhood obesity as a predictor of morbidity in adulthood: A systematic review and meta-analysis. *Obes. Rev.* **2016**, *17*, 56–67. [CrossRef]
8. Moral-Garcia, J.E.; Urchaga-Litago, J.D.; Ramos-Morcillo, A.J.; Maneiro, R. Relationship of parental support on healthy habits, school motivations and academic performance in adolescents. *Int. J. Environ. Res. Public Health* **2020**, *17*, 882. [CrossRef]
9. Sember, V.; Morrison, S.A.; Jurak, G.; Kovac, M.; Golobic, M.; Pavletic Samardzija, P.; Gabrijelcic, M.; Primozic, M.; Kotar, T.; Djomba, J.K.; et al. Results from Slovenia's 2018 report card on physical activity for children and youth. *J. Phys. Act. Health* **2018**, *15*, S404–S405. [CrossRef]
10. Yang, X.; Lee, J.; Gu, X.; Zhang, X.; Zhang, T. Physical fitness promotion among adolescents: Effects of a jump rope-based physical activity afterschool program. *Children* **2020**, *7*, 95. [CrossRef]
11. Taylor, S.L.; Noonan, R.J.; Knowles, Z.R.; McGrane, B.; Curry, W.B.; Fairclough, S.J. Acceptability and feasibility of single-component primary school physical activity interventions to inform the AS:Sk project. *Children* **2018**, *5*, 171. [CrossRef] [PubMed]
12. Duberg, A.; Moller, M.; Sunvisson, H. "I feel free": Experiences of a dance intervention for adolescent girls with internalizing problems. *Int. J. Qual. Stud. Health Well Being* **2016**, *11*, 31946. [CrossRef] [PubMed]
13. Sheppard, A.; Broughton, M.C. Promoting wellbeing and health through active participation in music and dance: A systematic review. *Int. J. Qual. Stud. Health Well Being* **2020**, *15*, 1732526. [CrossRef] [PubMed]
14. King, A.K.; McGill-Meeks, K.; Beller, J.P.; Burt Solorzano, C.M. Go girls!-Dance-based fitness to increase enjoyment of exercise in girls at risk for PCOS. *Children* **2019**, *6*, 99. [CrossRef]
15. Vassallo, A.J.; Hiller, C.; Stamatakis, E.; Pappas, E. Epidemiology of dance-related injuries presenting to emergency departments in the United States, 2000–2013. *Med. Probl. Perform. Art.* **2017**, *32*, 170–175. [CrossRef] [PubMed]
16. Ursej, E.; Zaletel, P. Injury occurrence in modern and hip-hop dancers: A systematic literature review. *Zdr. Varst.* **2020**, *59*, 195–201. [CrossRef] [PubMed]

17. Ursej, E.; Sekulic, D.; Prus, D.; Gabrilo, G.; Zaletel, P. Investigating the prevalence and predictors of injury occurrence in competitive hip hop dancers: Prospective analysis. *Int. J. Environ. Res. Public Health* **2019**, *16*, 3214. [CrossRef]
18. Jacobs, C.L.; Hincapie, C.A.; Cassidy, J.D. Musculoskeletal injuries and pain in dancers: A systematic review update. *J. Danc. Med. Sci.* **2012**, *16*, 74–84.
19. Hincapie, C.A.; Morton, E.J.; Cassidy, J.D. Musculoskeletal injuries and pain in dancers: A systematic review. *Arch. Phys. Med. Rehabil.* **2008**, *89*, 1819–1829. [CrossRef]
20. Kenny, S.J.; Palacios-Derflingher, L.; Shi, Q.; Whittaker, J.L.; Emery, C.A. Association between previous injury and risk factors for future injury in preprofessional ballet and contemporary dancers. *Clin. J. Sport Med.* **2019**, *29*, 209–217. [CrossRef]
21. van Winden, D.; Van Rijn, R.M.; Richardson, A.; Savelsbergh, G.J.P.; Oudejans, R.R.D.; Stubbe, J.H. Detailed injury epidemiology in contemporary dance: A 1-year prospective study of 134 students. *BMJ Open Sport Exerc. Med.* **2019**, *5*, e000453. [CrossRef] [PubMed]
22. Lee, L.; Reid, D.; Cadwell, J.; Palmer, P. Injury incidence, dance exposure and the use of the movement competency screen (Mcs) to identify variables associated with injury in full-time pre-professional dancers. *Int. J. Sports Phys. Ther.* **2017**, *12*, 352–370. [PubMed]
23. Ojofeitimi, S.; Bronner, S.; Woo, H. Injury incidence in hip hop dance. *Scand. J. Med. Sci. Sports* **2012**, *22*, 347–355. [CrossRef] [PubMed]
24. Luke, A.C.; Kinney, S.A.; D. Hemecourt, P.A.; Baum, J.; Owen, M.; Micheli, L.J. Determinants of injuries in young dancers. *Med. Probl. Perform. Artist.* **2002**, *17*, 105–112.
25. Zaletel, P.; Sekulic, D.; Zenic, N.; Esco, M.R.; Sajber, D.; Kondric, M. The association between body-built and injury occurrence in pre-professional ballet dancers—Separated analysis for the injured body-locations. *Int. J. Occup. Med. Environ. Health* **2017**, *30*, 151–159. [CrossRef] [PubMed]
26. Jubb, C.; Bell, L.; Cimelli, S.; Wolman, R. Injury patterns in hip hop dancers. *J. Dance Med. Sci.* **2019**, *23*, 145–149. [CrossRef]
27. Premelč, J.; Vučković, G.; James, N.; Dimitriou, L. A Retrospective investigation on age and gender differences of injuries in dance sport. *Int. J. Environ. Res. Public Health* **2019**, *16*, 4164. [CrossRef]
28. Hrysomallis, C. Relationship between balance ability, training and sports injury risk. *Sports Med.* **2007**, *37*, 547–556. [CrossRef]
29. Steinberg, N.; Siev-Ner, I.; Peleg, S.; Dar, G.; Masharawi, Y.; Zeev, A.; Hershkovitz, I. Injury patterns in young, non-professional dancers. *J. Sports Sci.* **2011**, *29*, 47–54. [CrossRef]
30. Aandstad, A.; Holtberget, K.; Hageberg, R.; Holme, I.; Anderssen, S.A. Validity and reliability of bioelectrical impedance analysis and skinfold thickness in predicting body fat in military personnel. *Mil. Med.* **2014**, *179*, 208–217. [CrossRef]
31. McLester, C.N.; Nickerson, B.S.; Kliszczewicz, B.M.; McLester, J.R. Reliability and agreement of various inbody body composition analyzers as compared to dual-energy X-ray absorptiometry in healthy men and women. *J. Clin. Densitom.* **2018**, *23*. [CrossRef] [PubMed]
32. Ambegaonkar, J.P.; Cortes, N.; Caswell, S.V.; Ambegaonkar, G.P.; Wyon, M. Lower extremity hypermobility, but not core muscle endurance influences balance in female collegiate dancers. *Int. J. Sports Phys. Ther.* **2016**, *11*, 220–229.
33. Gribble, P.A.; Hertel, J.; Plisky, P. Using the star excursion balance test to assess dynamic postural-control deficits and outcomes in lower extremity injury: A literature and systematic review. *J. Athl. Train.* **2012**, *47*, 339–357. [CrossRef] [PubMed]
34. Powden, C.J.; Dodds, T.K.; Gabriel, E.H. The reliability of the star excursion balance test and lower quarter Y-balance test in healthy adults: A systematic review. *Int. J. Sports Phys. Ther.* **2019**, *14*, 683–694. [CrossRef] [PubMed]
35. Clarsen, B.; Ronsen, O.; Myklebust, G.; Florenes, T.W.; Bahr, R. The Oslo sports trauma research center questionnaire on health problems: A new approach to prospective monitoring of illness and injury in elite athletes. *Br. J. Sports Med.* **2014**, *48*, 754–760. [CrossRef] [PubMed]
36. de Rezende, A.; Sampaio II, L.H.F.; Bittar, A.J.; da Silva Hamu, T.C.D.; Wyon, M.A.; Formiga, C. The relationship between vitamin D levels, injury and muscle function in adolescent dancers. *Int. J. Sports Med.* **2020**, *41*, 360–364. [CrossRef]

37. Bronner, S.; McBride, C.; Gill, A. Musculoskeletal injuries in professional modern dancers: A prospective cohort study of 15 years. *J. Sports Sci.* **2018**, *36*, 1880–1888. [CrossRef]
38. Campoy, F.A.; Coelho, L.R.; Bastos, F.N.; Netto Júnior, J.; Vanderlei, L.C.; Monteiro, H.L.; Padovani, C.R.; Pastre, C.M. Investigation of risk factors and characteristics of dance injuries. *Clin. J. Sport Med.* **2011**, *21*, 493–498. [CrossRef]
39. Post, E.G.; Trigsted, S.M.; Riekena, J.W.; Hetzel, S.; McGuine, T.A.; Brooks, M.A.; Bell, D.R. The association of sport specialization and training volume with injury history in youth athletes. *Am. J. Sports Med.* **2017**, *45*, 1405–1412. [CrossRef]
40. Jacobs, C.L.; Cassidy, J.D.; Côté, P.; Boyle, E.; Ramel, E.; Ammendolia, C.; Hartvigsen, J.; Schwartz, I. Musculoskeletal injury in professional dancers: Prevalence and associated factors: An international cross-sectional study. *Clin. J. Sport Med.* **2017**, *27*, 153–160. [CrossRef]
41. Cho, C.H.; Song, K.S.; Min, B.W.; Lee, S.M.; Chang, H.W.; Eum, D.S. Musculoskeletal injuries in break-dancers. *Injury* **2009**, *40*, 1207–1211. [CrossRef] [PubMed]
42. Kauther, M.D.; Wedemeyer, C.; Wegner, A.; Kauther, K.M.; von Knoch, M. Breakdance injuries and overuse syndromes in amateurs and professionals. *Am. J. Sports Med.* **2009**, *37*, 797–802. [CrossRef] [PubMed]
43. Simmel, L. *Dance Medicine in Practice: Anatomy, Injury Prevention, Training*; Taylor and Francis: London, UK, 2013.
44. Han, J.; Anson, J.; Waddington, G.; Adams, R.; Liu, Y. The Role of ankle proprioception for balance control in relation to sports performance and injury. *Biomed. Res. Int* **2015**, *2015*, 842804. [CrossRef] [PubMed]
45. Lai, W.C.; Wang, D.; Chen, J.B.; Vail, J.; Rugg, C.M.; Hame, S.L. Lower quarter Y-balance test scores and lower extremity injury in NCAA division I athletes. *Orthop. J. Sports Med.* **2017**, *5*, 2325967117723666. [CrossRef]
46. Plisky, P.J.; Rauh, M.J.; Kaminski, T.W.; Underwood, F.B. Star excursion balance test as a predictor of lower extremity injury in high school basketball players. *J. Orthop. Sports Phys. Ther.* **2006**, *36*, 911–919. [CrossRef]
47. Smith, C.A.; Chimera, N.J.; Warren, M. Association of y balance test reach asymmetry and injury in division I athletes. *Med. Sci. Sports Exerc.* **2015**, *47*, 136–141. [CrossRef]
48. Brachman, A.; Kamieniarz, A.; Michalska, J.; Pawlowski, M.; Slomka, K.J.; Juras, G. Balance training programs in athletes—A systematic review. *J. Hum. Kinet.* **2017**, *58*, 45–64. [CrossRef]
49. Valovich McLeod, T.C. The effectiveness of balance training programs on reducing the incidence of ankle sprains in adolescent athletes. *J. Sport Rehabil.* **2008**, *17*, 316–323. [CrossRef]
50. Muehlbauer, T.; Wagner, V.; Brueckner, D.; Schedler, S.; Schwiertz, G.; Kiss, R.; Hagen, M. Effects of a blocked versus an alternated sequence of balance and plyometric training on physical performance in youth soccer players. *BMC Sports Sci. Med. Rehabil.* **2019**, *11*, 18. [CrossRef]
51. Gebel, A.; Lesinski, M.; Behm, D.G.; Granacher, U. Effects and dose-response relationship of balance training on balance performance in youth: A systematic review and meta-analysis. *Sports Med.* **2018**, *48*, 2067–2089. [CrossRef]

Publisher's Note: MDPI stays neutral with regard to jurisdictional claims in published maps and institutional affiliations.

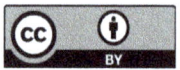

© 2020 by the authors. Licensee MDPI, Basel, Switzerland. This article is an open access article distributed under the terms and conditions of the Creative Commons Attribution (CC BY) license (http://creativecommons.org/licenses/by/4.0/).

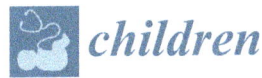

Communication

Optimum Angle of Force Production Temporarily Changes Due to Growth in Male Adolescence

Junya Saeki [1,2,*], Satoshi Iizuka [1], Hiroaki Sekino [3], Ayahiro Suzuki [3], Toshihiro Maemichi [3] and Suguru Torii [1]

1. Faculty of Sport Sciences, Waseda University, 2-579-15 Mikajima, Tokorozawa, Saitama 359-1192, Japan; anporian@gmail.com (S.I.); shunto@waseda.jp (S.T.)
2. Japan Society for the Promotion of Science, 5-3-1 Kojimachi, Chiyoda-ku, Tokyo 102-0083, Japan
3. Graduate School of Sport Sciences, Waseda University, 2-579-15 Mikajima, Tokorozawa, Saitama 359-1192, Japan; ry52112049@gmail.com (H.S.); sumanana-107@akane.waseda.jp (A.S.); t.m.waseda@ruri.waseda.jp (T.M.)
* Correspondence: saeki.junya.55z@kyoto-u.jp

Received: 1 December 2020; Accepted: 1 January 2021; Published: 3 January 2021

Abstract: The peak increase in lean mass in adolescents is delayed from peak height velocity (PHV), and muscle flexibility temporarily decreases as bones grow. If the decrease in muscle flexibility is caused by muscle elongation, the relationship between the exerted torque and the joint angle could change in adolescents. The purpose of this study was to investigate the change in the optimum angle of force production due to growth. Eighty-eight healthy boys were recruited for this study. Isokinetic knee extension muscle strength of the dominant leg was recorded. The outcome variable was the knee flexion angle when maximal knee extension torque was produced (optimum angle). The age at which PHV occurred was estimated from subjects' height history. We calculated the difference between the age at measurement and the expected age of PHV (growth age). A regression analysis was performed with the optimal angle of force exertion as the dependent variable and the growth age as the independent variable. Then, a polynomial formula with the lowest *p*-value was obtained. A significant cubic regression was obtained between optimum angle and growth age. The results suggest that the optimum angle of force production temporarily changes in male adolescence.

Keywords: force–angle relationship; isokinetic muscle strength; muscle–tendon unit; maximal voluntary contraction; growth spurt; children

1. Introduction

The incidence of sports injuries in adolescents increases until 15 to 16 years of age and decreases thereafter [1,2]. The cause has been considered to be influenced by bone mineral density (BMD) because the whole body BMD of the adolescent decreases when peak bone length increases, and many distal radius fractures occur at this time [3]. However, while whole body BMD recovers after its lowest point at around 13 years, also the time of peak height velocity (PHV) [3], the incidence of sports injury increases until 15 to 16 years of age [1]. Thus, it is not possible to explain the cause of the high incidence of sports injuries in adolescents from BMD only.

The lean mass peak increase in adolescents is delayed from PHV [4], and muscle flexibility temporarily decreases with increasing bone length [5,6]. A previous study on the tibialis anterior of rabbits showed that the exerted force changed the muscle elongation when the tibia was cut and the bone was torn in the longitudinal direction [7]. Because muscle length is changed by the joint angle [8], the exerted muscle force is changed by a joint angle (force–angle relationship) [9]. A previous study in vivo reported that the peak torque of the isokinetic contraction did not change, but the peak angle was changed by a chronic static stretching program [10]. As such, it was suggested that the force–angle relationship may be related to the change of muscle flexibility. Considering the above background, the relationships between exerted torque and joint angle may change during the muscle elongation period when bone growth precedes muscle growth. If the force–angle relationship temporarily changes in an adolescent, it could affect body control and the occurrence of sports injuries. However, change in the force–angle relationship has not been investigated.

To prevent sports injuries in adolescents, further understanding of the force production characteristics is necessary. Therefore, the purpose of this study was to investigate the relationship between the optimum angle of force production and growth age. The muscle flexibility temporarily decreases during adolescence [5,6], which could lead to muscle elongation and a temporary change in the force–angle relationship. We hypothesized that the optimum angle of force production changes curvilinearly during adolescence.

2. Materials and Methods

2.1. Subjects

Eighty-eight healthy junior high school boys (age: 13.6 ± 1.0 years, height: 157.9 ± 9.2 cm, body mass: 47.1 ± 8.8 kg; means ± SDs) were recruited in this study. The inclusion criteria were male junior high school soccer players who participated in a medical examination in their team. Exclusion criteria included history of lower extremity orthopedic surgeries or orthopedic disorders in the lower extremities on measurement day. Written informed consent was obtained from parents of the subjects prior to participation. This study was approved by an institutional human research ethics committee (2013-167) and was carried out in accordance with the declaration of Helsinki.

2.2. Measurement of the Optimum Angle

Isokinetic knee extension muscle strength of the dominant leg was recorded using an electric dynamometer (BIODEX System 3, BIODEX, Shirley, NY, USA). The subjects were seated on the dynamometer with their trunk, pelvic, and dominant thigh secured to a dynamometer by using non-elastic straps. The subjects' dominant leg was secured to an attachment and rotation axis of the knee joint was matched with the rotation axis of the dynamometer in a drooped position of the leg. The angle at which the thigh and leg of the subject were perpendicular was set as 90° of the dynamometer. At the measurement, the maximal isokinetic contraction of the knee extension was conducted at 60°/s in the range of maximal knee flex position to maximal knee extension position. The measurement was taken 3 times. We calculated the average value of the maximal knee extension torque (peak torque). The optimal angle of the force production was calculated by imposing the obtained scatter diagram of the joint angle and the exerted torque with a cubic curve and obtaining the coordinates of the local maximum point.

2.3. Estimation of the Growth Age

To calculate the subjects PHV age, height history in primary school was determined by listing annual physical measurement data on a questionnaire. In addition, the subjects' height in junior high school was recorded using a height meter. PHV age was estimated from the acquired height history using analysis software (AUXAL 3.1, Scientific Software International, Skokie, IL, USA). Finally, we calculated the difference between age at measurement and PHV, as a growth age.

2.4. Statistics

Descriptive data are presented as means ± SDs. Statistical analyses were performed using statistical software (SPSS Statistics 26; IBM, Chicago, IL, USA). To investigate the development of the peak torque, a linear regression analysis was performed with the peak torque as the dependent variable and the growth age as the independent variable. Subsequently, to investigate the development of the optimum angle, a regression analysis was performed with the optimal angle of force exertion as the dependent variable and the growth age as the independent variable. In these analyses, a polynomial formula with the lowest p-value was obtained. For all tests, the statistical significance was set at $p < 0.05$.

3. Results

The PHV age and the growth age were 13.3 ± 0.9 and 0.3 ± 1.5 years, respectively. A significant linear regression was obtained between the peak torque and growth age ($p < 0.001$, $R^2 = 0.40$) (Figure 1). A significant cubic regression was obtained between optimum angle and growth age ($p = 0.01$, $R^2 = 0.14$) (Figure 2). Coordinates of the minimal local value and maximal local value were (−1.0, 67.6) and (2.3, 74.6), respectively.

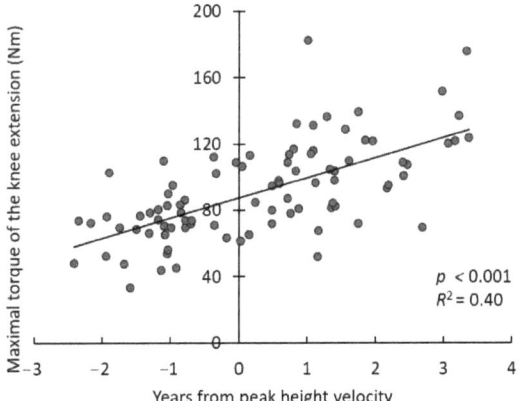

Figure 1. Relationships between maximal torque of knee extension and growth age.

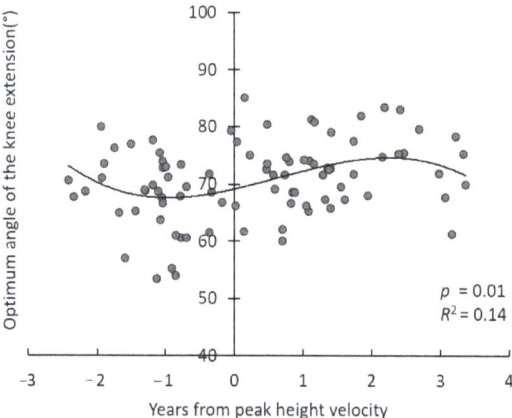

Figure 2. Relationships between optimum angle of the knee extension and growth age.

4. Discussion

The present study investigated the relationship between the optimum angle of force production and growth age. The main finding of the present study was that the relationship between the optimum angle and growth age was regressed by a cubic curve. To the best of our knowledge, this is the first study investigating the change in the optimum angle of force production during growth.

The PHV age was 13.3 ± 0.9 in this study and this result was the same as that reported by a previous study for Japanese subjects [11]. However, the PHV age was 0.2 to 0.8 years earlier than previous studies for Europeans and North Americans [4,12,13]. It is considered that race might influence the inter-study differences in PHV age.

A significant linear regression relationship was obtained between the peak torque and growth age. The relationship between optimum angle and growth age was significant when analyzed using the cubic regression model. These results support our hypothesis, and suggest that the optimum angle temporarily changes, despite the peak torque of force production developed with growth. The optimum angle of knee extension force production was temporarily smaller at approximately 1 year before PHV because the growth age on the minimal local value was −1.0 years. According to previous studies, it is reported that the increase in femur length of male adolescent peaks at 1.1 years before PHV [14]. The growth age when the optimum angle reaches its minimal value in this study nearly coincided with the increase in femur length in the previous study. In addition, it has been reported in other studies of the Japanese population that the flexibility of the quadriceps femoris muscle decreases in around 12-year-old individuals [5]. The optimum angle of force production in the present study was shown to be the minimum local around 12 years old when converted to age. Considering this, the increase of bone length and decrease of muscle flexibility could be related to temporary changes of the optimum angle of the knee extension muscle force production.

The results of the present study showed that the optimum angle of knee extension muscle force production temporarily decreases with growth. The muscle lengthens by an increase in bone length [7], and muscle length (joint angle) affects the force production [9,15]. Therefore, muscle elongation due to an increase of bone length could affect the force–angle relationship. In particular, because the quadriceps femoris muscle is elongated when the knee is flexed, muscle elongation due to growth is considered to cause the same change as knee flexion. Based on the above, the optimum angle of knee extension force production was considered to temporarily decrease due to growth.

The growth age of the maximum local value on the regression curve was 2.3 years. The peak of the temporary decrease in BMD was almost the same as that of PHV [3], which was earlier than the timing at which the optimum angle became the original value after the temporary change. In addition, because the average PHV age was 13.3 years, the optimum angle of force production was shown to be a maximum local at 15 to 16 years old when converted to age. In a previous study in Europeans and North Americans, the incidence of sports injuries in adolescents increased until 15 to 16 years of age and decreased after this period [1,2]. Although the PHV age in the present study was 0.2 to 0.8 years earlier than previous studies for Europeans and North Americans [4,12,13], the maximum local of the optimum was just before or almost the same as the timing when the incidence of sports injury begins to decline. Therefore, adolescent sports injuries could be affected by changes in force production characteristics due to growth.

There are a few limitations in this study. First, because the knee joint angle during force production was not measured, the joint angle in this study is different from the actual joint angle. Therefore, we do not mention the specific joint angle. However, the knee joint angle was defined using the same method in all subjects. Thus, this limitation cannot affect the result that the optimum angle of force production changes due to growth in adolescents. Second, because the range of the subjects' age was limited, it is not clear when the change of the optimal angle begins. A previous study showed that the muscle flexibility of the quadriceps muscle decreased in boys aged 11 years [5]. In addition, there is a sex difference in the incidence of Osgood–Schlatter disease, which is related to the quadricep muscle flexibility [16,17]. Therefore, further research needs to include at least 11-year-old boys and investigate the sex difference of the optimum angle change.

5. Conclusions

This study investigated the change in the optimum angle of knee extension force production due to growth. The results showed that the optimal angle is temporarily changed to the loose position of the quadriceps femoris muscle at approximately the same time as the increase in femur length in a previous study, and returned to the original within a few years. This suggests that the force–angle relationship temporarily changes with muscle elongation due to skeletal growth.

Author Contributions: Conceptualization, J.S. and T.M.; methodology, J.S.; formal analysis, J.S.; data curation, J.S. and A.S.; writing—original draft preparation, J.S.; writing—review and editing, S.T.; supervision, S.T.; project administration, S.I., H.S. and S.T.; funding acquisition, J.S. All authors have read and agreed to the published version of the manuscript.

Funding: This research was funded by a Grant-in-Aid from the Japan Society for the Promotion of Science Fellows (18J01881).

Institutional Review Board Statement: The study was conducted according to the guidelines of the Declaration of Helsinki, and approved by the Ethics Review Committee on Human Research of Waseda University (2013-167).

Informed Consent Statement: Informed consent was obtained from all subjects involved in the study.

Data Availability Statement: The data presented in this study are available on request from the corresponding author.

Acknowledgments: We appreciate Shinoda for helping in recruitment.

Conflicts of Interest: The authors declare no conflict of interest.

References

1. Bruhmann, B.; Schneider, S. Risk groups for sports injuries among adolescents—Representative German national data. *Child Care Health Dev.* **2011**, *37*, 597–605. [CrossRef] [PubMed]
2. McQuillan, R.; Campbell, H. Gender differences in adolescent injury characteristics: A population-based study of hospital A & E data. *Public Health* **2006**, *120*, 732–741. [CrossRef] [PubMed]
3. Faulkner, R.A.; Davison, K.S.; Bailey, D.A.; Mirwald, R.L.; Baxter-Jones, A.D. Size-corrected BMD decreases during peak linear growth: Implications for fracture incidence during adolescence. *J. Bone Min. Res.* **2006**, *21*, 1864–1870. [CrossRef] [PubMed]
4. Rauch, F.; Bailey, D.A.; Baxter-Jones, A.; Mirwald, R.; Faulkner, R. The 'muscle-bone unit' during the pubertal growth spurt. *Bone* **2004**, *34*, 771–775. [CrossRef] [PubMed]
5. Nakase, J.; Aiba, T.; Goshima, K.; Takahashi, R.; Toratani, T.; Kosaka, M.; Ohashi, Y.; Tsuchiya, H. Relationship between the skeletal maturation of the distal attachment of the patellar tendon and physical features in preadolescent male football players. *Knee Surg. Sports Traumatol. Arthrosc.* **2014**, *22*, 195–199. [CrossRef] [PubMed]
6. Yague, P.H.; De La Fuente, J.M. Changes in height and motor performance relative to peak height velocity: A mixed-longitudinal study of Spanish boys and girls. *Am. J. Hum. Biol.* **1998**, *10*, 647–660. [CrossRef]
7. Simpson, A.H.; Williams, P.E.; Kyberd, P.; Goldspink, G.; Kenwright, J. The response of muscle to leg lengthening. *J. Bone Jt. Surg. Br.* **1995**, *77*, 630–636. [CrossRef]
8. Refshauge, K.M.; Chan, R.; Taylor, J.L.; McCloskey, D.I. Detection of movements imposed on human hip, knee, ankle and toe joints. *Phys. Rev.* **1995**, *488*, 231–241. [CrossRef] [PubMed]
9. Williams, M.; Stutzman, L. Strength variation through the range of joint motion. *Phys. Ther. Rev.* **1959**, *39*, 145–152. [CrossRef] [PubMed]
10. Nakao, S.; Ikezoe, T.; Nakamura, M.; Umegaki, H.; Fujita, K.; Umehara, J.; Kobayashi, T.; Ibuki, S.; Ichihashi, N. Chronic Effects of a Static Stretching Program on Hamstring Strength. *J. Strength Cond. Res.* **2019**. [CrossRef] [PubMed]
11. Takei, S.; Taketomi, S.; Tanaka, S.; Torii, S. Growth pattern of lumbar bone mineral content and trunk muscles in adolescent male soccer players. *J. Bone Min. Metab.* **2020**, *38*, 338–345. [CrossRef] [PubMed]
12. Van der Sluis, A.; Elferink-Gemser, M.T.; Brink, M.S.; Visscher, C. Importance of peak height velocity timing in terms of injuries in talented soccer players. *Int. J. Sports Med.* **2015**, *36*, 327–332. [CrossRef] [PubMed]
13. Barbour-Tuck, E.; Erlandson, M.; Muhajarine, N.; Foulds, H.; Baxter-Jones, A. Longitudinal patterns in BMI and percent total body fat from peak height velocity through emerging adulthood into young adulthood. *Am. J. Hum. Biol.* **2018**, *30*. [CrossRef] [PubMed]
14. Smith, S.L.; Buschang, P.H. Longitudinal models of long bone growth during adolescence. *Am. J. Hum. Biol.* **2005**, *17*, 731–745. [CrossRef]
15. Gordon, A.M.; Huxley, A.F.; Julian, F.J. The variation in isometric tension with sarcomere length in vertebrate muscle fibres. *J. Physiol.* **1966**, *184*, 170–192. [CrossRef]
16. Ito, E.; Iwamoto, J.; Azuma, K.; Matsumoto, H. Sex-specific differences in injury types among basketball players. *Open Access J. Sports Med.* **2015**, *6*, 1–6. [CrossRef] [PubMed]
17. Nakase, J.; Goshima, K.; Numata, H.; Oshima, T.; Takata, Y.; Tsuchiya, H. Precise risk factors for Osgood-Schlatter disease. *Arch. Orthop. Trauma Surg.* **2015**, *135*, 1277–1281. [CrossRef]

Publisher's Note: MDPI stays neutral with regard to jurisdictional claims in published maps and institutional affiliations.

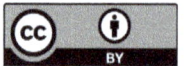

© 2021 by the authors. Licensee MDPI, Basel, Switzerland. This article is an open access article distributed under the terms and conditions of the Creative Commons Attribution (CC BY) license (http://creativecommons.org/licenses/by/4.0/).

MDPI
St. Alban-Anlage 66
4052 Basel
Switzerland
Tel. +41 61 683 77 34
Fax +41 61 302 89 18
www.mdpi.com

Children Editorial Office
E-mail: children@mdpi.com
www.mdpi.com/journal/children

www.ingramcontent.com/pod-product-compliance
Lightning Source LLC
LaVergne TN
LVHW070611100526
838202LV00012B/616